The Enchanted World of Sleep

# The Enchanted World of Sleep

PERETZ LAVIE

Translated by Anthony Berris

Yale University Press    New Haven and London

Published with assistance from the Kingsley Trust
Association Publication Fund established by the
Scroll and Key Society of Yale College.

First published in Hebrew in 1993 by Yedioth
Ahronoth Books; Chemed Books, P.P.B. 37744,
Tel Aviv 61356, Israel.

Designed by Sonia L. Scanlon.
Set in Bodoni type by Rainsford Type, Danbury,
Connecticut.
Printed in the United States of America by R. R.
Donnelley & Sons, Harrisonburg, Virginia.

Library of Congress Cataloging-in-Publication Data
Lavie, P. (Peretz), 1949–
 ['Olamah ha-kasum shel ha-shenah. English]
 The enchanted world of sleep / Peretz Lavie ;
translated by Anthony Berris.
  p. cm.
 Includes bibliographical references
 and index.
 ISBN 0-300-06602-3 (cloth:alk. paper)
 ISBN 0-300-07436-0 (pbk.:alk. paper)
 1. Sleep—Popular works. 2. Sleep
 disorders—Popular works.
 I. Title.
 QP425.L3713  1996
 612.8'21—dc20  95-41304
       CIP

A catalogue record for this book is available from
the British Library.

The paper in this book meets the guidelines for
permanence and durability of the Committee on
Production Guidelines for Book Longevity of the
Council on Library Resources.

10 9 8 7 6 5 4 3

*To Lena*
*who believed from the beginning*

# Contents

*Foreword by Michel Jouvet ix*

*Introduction xi*

1 Sleep and Death 1

2 Brain Waves 8

3 Nathaniel Kleitman 18

4 The Rhythm of Sleep 26

5 The Twenty-five Hour Day 35

6 From Sun Clocks to Biological Clocks 54

7 Dreams: Creatures of the Brain 65

8 Alfred Maury and the Dream of the Guillotine 76

9 Dreaming as a Separate Reality 89

10 Do Fish Dream? 98

11 The Need for Sleep 111

12 The Eccentricity of REM Sleep 129

13 Sleep Centers 151

14 Sleep Medicine: The First Steps 161

15 Treating Insomnia 174

16 The Physical and Medical Causes of Insomnia 184

17 Disorders in Sleep Timing 189

18 Children Who Refuse to Sleep 205

19 Excessive Sleepiness, or "In the Arms of Morpheus" 216

20 Narcolepsy: Reversal of the Natural Order 234

*Epilogue 243*

*References 247*

*Index 263*

# Foreword

Every night the story of sleep, which is as old as time itself, unfolds before us.

More than three billion years ago, evolution discovered the biological clock of blue-green algae, a clock which would force us to fall asleep in a regular cycle even if we were imprisoned forever in total isolation.

Some five hundred million years ago, during humankind's developmental process, the homeostatic mechanisms which prevent us from remaining awake for prolonged periods were created in the vertebrates. About two million years ago, neurobiological mechanisms helped create the dream condition which from that time on has played a major role in human culture.

It was the dream experience which evoked the assumption of duality between body and soul and which, apparently, became the catalyst for the creation of the concepts of "eternal life" and "God."

Finally, in 1879 Thomas Alva Edison invented the light bulb and became responsible, quite inadvertently, for the myriad discomforts which derive from the incompatibility between our sleeping time and the substitution of light for darkness. The various constraints which sometimes force us to remain awake at night are the root cause of the vexing divergence between the internal human clock, which continues to deny Edison, and the dictates of modern society. With extraordinary eloquence based upon a vast store of professional knowledge and innovative concepts of the physiology of sleep and dreams, among them that of the "forbidden zone for sleep," Peretz Lavie tells us the story of what is contained in a single night's sleep.

Although I am unable to summarize Lavie's contribution to

the study of sleep here, the opportunity I have been given in these few inadequate preparatory remarks are an expression of my great admiration for both this wonderful book and its author, who is one of the most talented pioneers in the study of sleep and dreams.

Michel Jouvet

# Introduction

In my various encounters with people, I am frequently asked the unavoidable question "What do you do?" and then find myself hesitating for a few seconds before replying, "I am engaged in the study of sleep."

My hesitation stems from the fact that experience has taught me that there are two responses to my reply. The first is usually accompanied by a burst of laughter: "The study of sleep? What needs to be studied about sleep?" This is usually followed by a reflex yawn, with which my questioner seems to be telling me, "I, too, study the subject occasionally."

The second response is a prompt request for advice and medication to combat snoring, insomnia, or other sleep-linked problems.

When my grandfather—a farmer who tilled the land with every fiber of his being—first heard that I intended to devote myself to the study of sleep, he tried to convince me to look for a more "useful" profession. "What can a man achieve in his life if he is occupied with sleep?" he argued vigorously.

It is sometimes difficult to convince people that sleep is an enthralling subject, but it is my hope that readers of this book will end up feeling as I do. I should point out that I came to the world of sleep almost by chance. For this I thank Prof. Zvi Giora of the Department of Psychology at the University of Tel Aviv, who encouraged me to enter the field, and Rotary International, which gave me a student grant to complete my doctorate at the sleep laboratories of the University of Florida under the guidance of Prof. Bernie Webb, one of the founders of modern sleep research.

In Webb's laboratory I learned the meaning of sleep research. I completed my post-doctoral studies at the University of California, San Diego, under the tutelage of Prof. Daniel

Kripke, and in 1975 I joined the Faculty of Medicine at the Technion—
Israel Institute of Technology in Haifa, of which I am now the Dean.

The Technion Sleep Laboratory has grown and developed into one
of the biggest research facilities of its kind in the world. Every night
about twenty people "enjoy" a stay in the laboratory with the sole objective of enabling us to discover the causes of their sleeping problems.

The laboratory's successful development must be ascribed, first and
foremost, to its devoted staff, who work literally day and night on clinical
work and research. Without their help, enthusiasm, and zeal, we never
would have achieved the high standard of results that we have. I extend
my heartfelt gratitude to all of them.

The Rigler-Deutsch Foundation has granted generous financial support to the Technion Sleep Laboratory, and Lloyd Rigler, a true human-
itarian and lover of humankind, has provided us with much advice, help,
and encouragement, for which we are indebted.

My thanks go, too, to Bernie Webb, Allan Rechtschaffen, Nathaniel
Kleitman, Jürgen Aschoff, Bill Dement, and Lev Mukhamatov, who all
graciously provided me with photographs from their collections. I am
grateful to Boehringer Ingelheim for permission to reproduce figures
4–7 and 9–11 in this book from its Postgraduate Medical Services series,
Sleep and Wakefulness. Bernie Webb, Allan Rechtschaffen, and Irene
Tobler also guided me with their excellent advice.

Special thanks are due to Michel Jouvet for the Foreword to this
book, to Anthony Berris for his excellent English translation, to Gay
Natanzon for the final preparation of the English version, and to Harry
Haskell of Yale University Press for the editing.

*The Enchanted World of Sleep* is written from my own personal viewpoint, and there may be a tendency—as frequently happens in such
cases—for the writer's role to be disproportionately emphasized. My aim
in writing this book was twofold. First, I have tried to describe the in-
credible evolution of a new area of scientific inquiry, to which I was a
privileged eyewitness. Second, I wanted to share my enthusiasm about
being involved in such an endeavor by describing some studies and findings from my own laboratory—even if they weren't always entirely original, or even of prime importance. I trust my fellow sleep researchers will
understand and forgive me.

The Enchanted World of Sleep

# Sleep and Death

Humans spend approximately one-third of their lives in sleep. Sleep does not discriminate between the African tribesman who lies down on his bed of dried leaves and the city dweller who retires to sleep on an expensive boxspring mattress in his high-rise apartment.

Sleep is common to all humankind—and humankind is equal before it. As the sun sets in China, more than a billion Chinese cover themselves with their blankets and lie down to sleep. A few hours later, in exactly the same way, Americans, too, will retire to sleep. However, all over the world there are people whose special duties oblige them to follow the reverse routine of waking up at night and sleeping during the day.

For thousands of years, sleep was viewed as an inseparable part of the order of nature, testimony to nature's good sense or the wisdom of the gods. No one was bothered by the question Why do we sleep? Sleep was the condition that separated the activities of one day from those of the next, and apart from dreaming, nothing of importance was considered to occur during those hours of oblivion. Dreaming was perceived not as a part of sleep but rather as the result of external influences exerted on the sleeper. Sleep was what happened between "Good evening" and "Good morning," but no more than that.

During the second half of the twentieth century, a revolution took place in the scientific approach to sleep. From a phenomenon of interest only to poets and philosophers, sleep became the subject of rigorous scientific research, utilizing advanced and innovative methods. Doctors, who had previously viewed sickness and disease as part of the awake and conscious human condition, and who had not considered it necessary to study sicknesses while their patients were asleep, began to realize that some ailments manifested themselves only when the patient was asleep.

The fact that sleep is unavoidable raises the possibility that it is something akin to short-term death. We can find a hint of this belief in the Jewish daily prayer book; every night before retiring, pious Jews entrust their souls to their Maker with the words "Blessed art thou, O Lord our God, King of the Universe, who makest the bands of sleep to fall upon mine eyes, and slumber upon mine eyelids. May it be thy will, O Lord my God and God of my fathers, to suffer me to lie down in peace and let me rise up again in peace." On awakening in the morning, they greet the Lord with the words "I give thanks unto thee, the living King, who restoreth my soul in compassion." Not only in Judaism is sleep viewed as a form of death; in Greek mythology, sleep (*hypnos*) and death (*thanatos*) are described as "twins of the night" who reside in the underworld.

Bernie Webb of the University of Florida, my first guide and mentor in the world of sleep, used to describe sleep as the "Gentle Tyrant," and indeed any choice between wakefulness and sleep is out of our hands. "Men and gods alike bowed to sleep in submission," said Homer in his *Iliad*. We are able to modify our eating and drinking habits to a great extent, but we can give up sleep only for short periods of time. There are those who succeed in changing their sexual habits completely, but the habit of sleeping is extremely difficult to change. A great many people would be prepared to pay a very high price for the ability to reduce their sleeping time—from, say, seven to three hours a night—but should they try, sleep would surely overtake them in a few days, thus adding its burden to their already semiclosed eyelids.

There can be no doubt that the sleep-wakefulness cycle is the most stable aspect of our behavior, endowing it with a regularity and a rhythm.

## VAPORS THAT RISE FROM THE STOMACH

Early scientific thought perceived sleep as a passive condition created by the isolation of the brain from the other parts of the body, and much evidence of this is to be found in ancient texts.

Alcmaeon, who lived in the sixth century B.C., claimed that sleep was caused by the blood receding from the blood vessels in the skin to the interior parts of the body, and awakening was caused by its return. The blood's disappearance from the skin caused immobility and an absence of sensation. Some saw sleep as a result of changes in the blood's characteristics and believed that a drop in blood temperature was the cause of sleep, while a rise caused wakefulness.

One of the first to devote systematic thought to sleep was Aristotle, who assembled his predictions and ideas in his work *De somno et vigilia* (On sleeping and waking). According to Aristotle, sleep and wakefulness are results of our ability to feel and comprehend the stimuli of our environment; ergo, sleep characterizes only those species which possess sensory organs. His description of the process of falling asleep is picturesque in the extreme. His theory suggests that while food is being digested, vapors rise from the stomach because of their higher temperature and collect in the head. As the brain cools, the vapors condense, flow downward, and then cool the heart. Aristotle, who perceived the heart as the body's sensory center, believed that its cooling was the cause and reason for sleep.

Greek philosophers and physicians agreed with Aristotle that isolation of the body from its senses was the cause of sleep, but unlike him they viewed the brain, not the heart, as the body's center of sensation. Socrates's pupil Plato and the eminent Greek physician Galen viewed the brain's isolation from the rest of the body, not the cooling of the heart, as the main reason for sleep. Like Aristotle, they believed that the causes of sleep were mechanical. Vapors rising from the stomach condensed on arrival at the brain, but instead of descending to the heart, as Aristotle believed, they blocked the brain's pores, thus isolating it from the rest of the body. And so, with his brain disconnected from his body, man slept.

Like other medical concepts, these concepts of sleep survived for more than fifteen hundred years. Changes introduced by physicians and philosophers during the Middle Ages, the Renaissance, and even later were minimal. Some claimed that the isolation of the brain from the body was not total, for sleep could be disturbed by loud noises or by shaking the sleeper. There were those who pinpointed the reason for sleep not in the entire brain but in a unique organ within it—the "common sensory" organ, to which, according to contemporary conventional wisdom, all bodily senses were linked. Some took the idea of vapors even further and claimed that sleep quality and duration were dependent upon the type and composition of the vapors which rose to the brain. Obviously, sleep was deep and especially long after a heavy meal, which would certainly produce a larger volume of vapors.

The Greek concept of vapors blocking the brain's pores and thereby causing sleep remained basically unchanged until relatively modern times. The only changes that the concept then underwent dealt with the reasons and factors behind the isolation of the brain from the body. The "stomach vapors" were replaced by other factors, such as the flow of blood to the brain. In the eighteenth and nineteenth centuries, there were two schools of thought: one claimed that sleep was caused by "anemia"—in other words, a lack of blood in the brain—while the other argued with no less vigor that sleep was caused by an excess of blood in the brain. Both camps based their claims on controlled observations, generally of human or animal brains which had been exposed during surgery or as a result of a skull wound. Those who claimed that lack of blood was the cause of sleep argued that when human beings were asleep, their brains were pallid and shrunken, while in a state of wakefulness the brain was engorged with blood and dark in color. In contrast, the excess-blood school claimed that the brains of sleeping human beings were protuberant and dark in color but were shrunken in a state of wakefulness. Both camps were, of course, unaware of the fact that the flow of cerebral blood is under the rigid control of the nervous system and remains constant in both wakefulness and sleep.

Still others claimed that the isolation of the brain from the body was the result of swelling of the thyroid gland in the neck or swelling of the lymph glands. Others went even further and perceived sleep as a result of a cessation of cerebral activity—a kind of "short-circuit" caused by a separation of the nerve cells. They likened the nerve cells to organisms resembling amoebae which were capable of moving to and from one another.

In the history of scientific thought about the causes of sleep, the theories regarding hypnotoxins, or sleep toxins, have a special place. These were toxins which poisoned the brain, thus causing sleep. They were the catabolic products of metabolic processes which occurred during wakefulness and which accumulated throughout the day, and when they reached critical proportions they caused sleep. This theory was first propounded in the nineteenth century, and "incontrovertible proof" of its soundness was provided by French researchers. They put dogs to sleep by injecting them with fluids taken from the brains of other dogs which had been deprived of sleep for a long period. They believed that the fluids taken from the wakeful dogs' brains contained an accumulation of a hypnotoxin which would cause sleep in the other dogs. This approach also had its supporters in the twentieth century.

Some researchers saw musculoskeletal and nervous system "fatigue" as the main cause of sleep. The foremost advocate of this approach was Nathaniel Kleitman, who is credited with the greatest discovery in the field of sleep research, "rapid eye movement (REM) sleep," a discovery which upset the apple cart of earlier scientific approaches to the subject. Like other researchers, Kleitman believed that sleep was the result of muscle and nervous system fatigue.

Ivan Pavlov, the Russian physiologist and Nobel Prize–winner for physiology and medicine, also claimed that sleep was a condition in which inhibition of the brain's activity was induced reflexively. It is reasonable to assume that his ideas regarding sleep were influenced by his work on the conditioned reflex.

Yet by the beginning of the twentieth century there were signs of newer approaches. Some claimed that just as there are brain centers which control speech, hearing, or vision, there is also a special center which controls sleep. Activation of this center was said to cause sleep, while cessation of its activity, or the activation of an adjoining center, caused wakefulness. This theory is linked to the name of Constantin von Economo and to the fearful effects of the epidemic of encephalitis lethargica, "sleeping sickness," which swept across the globe at the end of the First World War, leaving millions dead in its wake. The enthralling figure of von Economo and his discoveries are worthy of more than passing mention, and I shall expand on them later.

## TENNIS BALLS AND SEISMOGRAPHS

To comprehend the essence of sleep, we must study it objectively and precisely. Our assessment of sleep is unreliable, and sometimes surprisingly erroneous. Take the common example of awakening from a brief

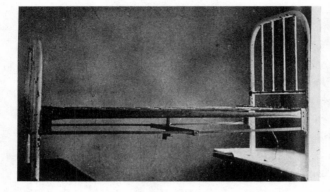

Fig. 1. A bed acti-meter used to investigate sleep in children. From S. Renshaw et al., *Children's Sleep* (New York: Macmillan, 1933), p. 38.

nap and feeling as though we have slept for hours. Conversely, there are those who awaken from eight or ten hours of sleep convinced that they have had only a brief nap, while others awaken from sleep which, to the observer, appeared to be deep and vehemently deny that they have been asleep at all. This inability to judge the length and depth of sleep is one of the principal assessment difficulties undergone by the patient suffering from a sleep disorder. Reliable and objective research methods are therefore required to "measure" sleep.

How, then, was sleep studied in the past? Early researchers observed natural phenomena, and their insights are still worthy of the highest praise. Consider this excerpt from Lucretius's essay on sensation and sex from *De rerum natura* (On the nature of the universe), written in the first century B.C.: "You will see mettlesome steeds, when their limbs are at rest, still continuing in sleep to sweat and pant as if straining all their strength to win the palm, or as if the lifted barriers of the starting-post had just released them. And the huntsman's hounds, while wrapped in gentle slumber, often toss their legs with a quick jerk and utter sudden whines and draw rapid breaths of air into their nostrils as if they were hot on a newly-found scent" (trans. R. E. Latham). Lucretius's description of a dog's dream sleep, distinguished as it is by much physical activity, is very accurate indeed.

But how could one measure phenomena such as the time it takes to fall asleep, which cannot be observed accurately? One of the methods used was to put an article, such as a stone or a small ball, into the sub-

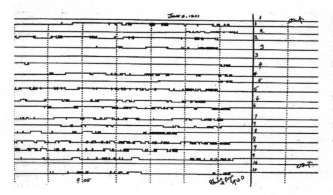

Fig. 2. A typical record of bed movements during the first hour of sleep. From S. Renshaw et al., *Children's Sleep* (New York: Macmillan, 1933), p. 49.

ject's hand and ask him or her to hold it outside the blankets. The moment the article fell from the hand as a result of muscle laxity was determined to be the moment of falling asleep. In other words, the fact that sleep caused muscle laxity was used to separate sleep from wakefulness.

One of the most popular methods of distinguishing between sleep and wakefulness was to measure body movements. Sleeping humans make almost no movement at all. The first instrument to record body movement continuously while the subject was asleep was invented by a German researcher called Szymanski. The instrument resembled a seismograph, connected either to the bed or to the subject's feet, which recorded even the smallest movement of the sleeper's body. The time of falling asleep was determined from the time that movement of the bed ceased. Thus it was also possible to measure the tranquility of sleep, the difference between the sleep of men and women, and how sleep was affected by drinking coffee, physical exertion, and other factors.

The bed-movement actimeter has been used in sleep research, mainly with children, since the beginning of the twentieth century. Today, however, the meter is very small and attached to the subject's wrist. Tremendous technical advances allow the storing of vast amounts of information on a subject's hand movements over a period of days, even months, in an instrument the size of an average wristwatch. Using a computer, the variations in the subject's hand movements are translated into minutes of sleep and wakefulness.

# Brain Waves

The most significant change in sleep research in particular and the study of the nervous system in general occurred with the discovery of brain waves and the advent of the electroencephalogram.

The idea that the nervous system was electrically active was first aired at the end of the eighteenth century. Luigi Galvani of Bologna was the first to demonstrate that the electrical stimulation of an exposed nerve caused contraction of the muscle to which the nerve was connected. His experiments on nerve stimulation in frogs have since become part of the bedrock of science. It later became apparent that electrical stimulation of various areas of the brain caused movements in different parts of the body; in fact, electrical stimulation was used to map the brain. From there it was a short road to demonstrating the connection between variations in electrical voltage on a nerve's surface and its activation.

The British researcher Richard Caton was the first scientifically to examine whether, by using electrical tracing of the brain's surface, it was possible to prove the activity of nerve centers beneath the trace electrodes. In 1875 Caton discovered that by placing electrodes over the surface of the area of the brain that is linked to vision, he could, by flashing a light into the eyes of a subject animal, detect variations in voltage. His findings also showed spontaneous variations in electrical activity, but he attached no special significance to this. At almost the same time a Polish scientist, Adolph Beck, conducted similar experiments and reached the same conclusions. Beck summed up his findings regarding spontaneous activity on the brain's surface thus (as cited in Brazier's *History of the Electrical Activity of the Brain*): "Even in the very first experiment I noticed—and repeated experiments all confirmed it—that the difference in potential between the electrodes when applied to two given points on the cortex of the hemispheres was not a stable level of potential; there was a continuous waxing and waning variation taking place which neither was related to the respiratory rhythm nor was it synchronous with the pulse, nor finally was it in any way dependent on movement of the animal, since it was present in curarized dogs. I therefore believe that these variations were the result of spontaneous activity in the brain centers."

Fifty years after Caton and Beck made their respective discoveries, which had resulted from experiments on animals, came conclusive proof that spontaneous electrical activity was indeed produced in the human brain. A German psychiatrist named Hans Berger, who worked at the Jena Psychiatric Hospital, discovered that electrical activity in the human brain could be traced over the surface of the skull. Berger began to investigate electrical activity of the brain following his study of parapsychological phenomena like telepathy and telekinesis. He claimed that it could be assumed that electrical activity of the brain could be traced during telepathic activity. After a year of experimentation, he succeeded in recording spontaneous electrical activity on the surface of the brain and gave it the name "encephalogram." He proved that electrical activity was reduced when the subject's sensations were exposed to stimulus or when the subject's mental processes were active. Berger shrouded his experiments in secrecy; entry to his laboratory was forbidden and he did not discuss his findings with any of his colleagues. His first published work on electrical activity in the brain appeared in 1929, five years after his first experiment. From that time on he published an additional article annually until 1934. The Nazis dismissed him from his post as director of the Jena Psychiatric Hospital in 1938, and three years later he was committed to a mental hospital in a state of depression. As a psychiatrist he found it difficult to come to terms with his own mental state and took his own life by hanging himself. Thus came to a tragic end the life of a man whose discoveries had completely changed scientific study of the brain. Today, one cannot imagine how it would be possible to diagnose nervous disorders or conduct scientific research on brain activity without tracing its electrical activity.

Discovery of the electrical activity of the brain opened new vistas on the study of sleep. Instead of recording bed movements or waiting for a

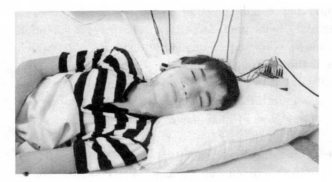

Fig. 3. A patient in
the Technion Sleep
Laboratory.

tennis ball to fall from the subject's hand, it became possible to attach
electrodes to the subject's head and record the spontaneous variations
taking place in the brain during the transition between sleep and wakefulness. I am convinced that early researchers who recorded the electrical
activity of the brain during this period were astounded when the electro-
magnetic pen first recorded a sleeping subject's brain waves. It is entirely
possible that they rushed to check that their instruments were in full
working order, for the difference between the activity of the sleeping and
wakeful brains is vast.

## WHAT IS TESTED IN THE SLEEP LABORATORY?

Modern sleep research is conducted principally in a sleep laboratory,
where electrophysiological recordings depicting the course of sleep are
made. These are called polysomnographic recordings. Apart from the
attachment of recording electrodes to the subject, sleeping conditions in
the laboratory differ little from those in his or her home. The bedrooms,
which are private, comfortable, and air-conditioned, are connected to the
adjoining control room, where the "sleep technicians" are on duty
throughout the night.

Three data sources provide reliable information on the process of
falling asleep and the changes which occur during sleep itself: brain
waves, eyeball movements, and muscle tonus.

Brain waves are recorded through electrodes attached to the subject's
head. The electrodes for recording eyeball movements are taped to the

head at either side of the eyes, while muscle tonus is usually recorded from the neck or chin muscles. The electrodes are connected to an amplifier located in the control room.

The moment a subject hears about the preparations involved in recording his or her sleep, the first question is always, "Will I be able to sleep with all those electrodes attached to my head?" The reply usually causes some surprise: not only can you actually sleep in the laboratory, but many people who suffer from severe and longstanding sleep-related disorders do so much faster, and sleep much more soundly, than they do in their own beds. As of this writing, more than fifteen thousand people, young and old, have spent a night in the Technion Sleep Laboratory. Some had problems falling asleep, while others had difficulty staying awake, but the total number of people who were actually unable to fall asleep in the laboratory does not exceed ten! The majority fall asleep within ten to fifteen minutes. How can someone bitterly complaining of insomnia manage to fall asleep so quickly, especially when festooned with electrodes? Possible answers to this question will be examined in Chapter 14.

Many people suffer from breathing problems or heart dysfunction while asleep. Therefore, in addition to our standard procedures, the following are also recorded: respiratory movements, air flow through the nose and mouth, blood oxygenation level, heart rate, and leg movements. If automatic behavior during sleep, such as sleepwalking or night terrors, is suspected, a continuous video film, using infrared light in order not to disturb the subject, is shot throughout the night. Watching a movie of this kind (lasting seven hours!) is not terribly exciting, but the findings are often of immeasurable importance.


FALLING ASLEEP

As early as 1935, when the first sleep recordings were conducted at Harvard University, it was clear that a gradual change in the electrical activity of the brain takes place during the transition from wakefulness to sleep. During wakefulness brain waves are extremely rapid; they occur at a rate of more than fifteen waves per second and are characterized by a very low voltage. As the level of alertness increases and the attention level intensifies, brain waves (known as beta waves) become more rapid and their voltage diminishes. An initial change in the brain's activity in preparation for sleep takes place during wakefulness, just before falling asleep.

Once the lights are off and the subject is comfortably settled, the electrical activity of his brain changes—especially if he closes his eyes. The rapid, low-voltage electrical activity that prevailed in his brain during periods of increased alertness is replaced by slower activity of some eight to ten waves per second. These are called alpha waves and have a higher voltage than those active during tense wakefulness. One of the identifying characteristics of alpha waves is their regular configuration, which resembles the teeth of a comb. In fact, they are sometimes so regular that it is difficult to believe that they were produced by a human brain and not an electronic instrument. Opening of the eyes or any other disturbance of the tranquil condition causes an immediate disappearance of the alpha waves and a reappearance of the beta waves indicating tense wakefulness. Alpha waves were previously known as "Berger waves" after the man who first succeeded in recording them, Hans Berger.

As they are directly connected to a relaxed state, alpha waves gained a great deal of popularity. The 1960s and 1970s saw the advent of an entire industry devoted to the production of electronic instruments which allowed the control of alpha waves using biological feedback techniques that "taught" people to relax. Researchers claimed that acquiring the ability to create alpha waves voluntarily would bring about a state of relaxation. Since tension was implicated in some psychosomatic illnesses such as hypertension and headaches, people who were unable to relax using traditional methods were encouraged to try "biofeedback" to control their alpha activity. But their high expectations were followed by great disappointment, for although many studies clearly proved that control of alpha waves could be achieved, there was no solid proof that it made any real contribution to health improvement.

The change from rapid, low-voltage beta waves to the more regular alpha waves takes place when subjects reduce their tension, close their eyes, and calm down. With people who are extremely tired or who have just returned home from a late-night party, this stage of serene and calm wakefulness with its expectation of sleep can continue for a minute or two, but with those who suffer problems in falling asleep, it can continue

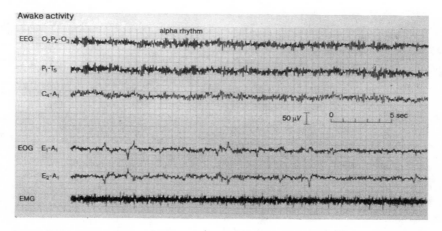

Fig. 4. Wakefulness: alpha waves

for an hour or more. The precise moment of falling asleep is most elusive. It is very difficult to pinpoint it by recording brain waves, for in most cases the change in brain waves while the subject moves from a condition of calm wakefulness to sleep is gradual and can last for several minutes. On condition that the process is allowed to continue undisturbed, the intense activity of the alpha waves will slowly be replaced by less rapid waves at a frequency of four to seven waves per second. These are called theta waves, and their amplitude is similar to that of alpha waves. In many cases, the changeover between the alpha and theta waves takes several minutes, and the impression given on the recording sheet is that of two opposing forces fighting for a foothold in the brain. Not without good reason is this stage called "sleep stage 1," "half sleep," or the "transitional stage."

In addition to the changes that occur in the brain waves, falling asleep is accompanied by other physiological changes, the most important of which occur in the skeletal and eye muscles, breathing movements, and pulse rate. In a state of wakefulness, muscle tonus allows us, among other things, to hold our heads up, but the skeletal muscles relax as we fall asleep. One result of this relaxation is "nodding off," which sometimes occurs, for example, during a long, boring meeting. When someone falls asleep while in a sitting position, relaxation of the neck muscles causes the head to fall forward onto the chest, and the resultant

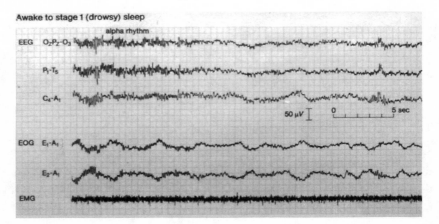

' Fig. 5. Falling asleep: transition from wakefulness to sleep stage 1

sudden blow of chin on chest wakes the sleeper up abruptly, his head straightens up momentarily, and the process is then repeated. Hence the quaint description of this activity: to the observer, the sleeper is "nodding."

The muscle relaxation that signifies falling asleep is sometimes interrupted by a sudden start called a "hypnic jerk" for which we have no well-established explanation, although we may assume that it results from a change in the brain to decrease muscle tonus. Like the sudden forward jump a car makes after a clumsy gear change, this could cause an "error" in the activation of a group of muscles, thus resulting in a sudden start. The effects of hypnic jerk are short-term and the sleeper immediately returns to a half-asleep condition. Together with relaxation of the skeletal muscles, stabilization of breathing movements and heart rate also occurs. Breathing depth is reduced and it is sometimes difficult to observe breathing movements at all. A great change occurs in eye muscle activity. In a state of wakefulness, we comb our immediate surroundings looking for objects and images with incessant, rapid, coordinated eye movements. In the falling asleep stage, these eye movements, which are mainly lateral (from right to left and left to right) give way to slow, more cumbersome, and recurring vertical movements. These slow eye movements are most easily observed in infants, who sleep with their eyes half-open. In the falling asleep stage, we can see that the infants' eyeballs disappear for

short periods to be replaced by the whites of the eyes, the vertical movement having moved the eyeballs in an upward direction. After falling
asleep, the eye movements disappear, only to reappear about an hour
and a half later in a totally different form.

## THE K-COMPLEX AND SLEEP SPINDLES

So when can we say with certainty that someone has fallen asleep? It is
difficult to judge by the appearance of the eyes alone; anyone familiar
with movies or the theater knows that faking sleep is a relatively easy
matter. The impression would be conveyed if someone simply lay motionless and closed his eyes for a few minutes. Even brain waves showing
continuous theta activity do not guarantee that someone has indeed fallen
asleep. If during the immobile condition of continuous theta activity we
were to nudge a group of sleepers and ask them if they were asleep, half
would say yes and the remainder would deny it. Many people are capable
of continuous attention to their surroundings and of immediate response,
even when the electrical activity of their brain is that of theta waves. This
explains why this stage is called half sleep. Additional physiological
indications are necessary in order to determine with any degree of certainty if the subject is indeed asleep.

These indications are provided by two further brain waves which
appear only in the sleeping brain: K-complexes and sleep spindles. The
K-complex is a single high-amplitude wave, some four times stronger
than the background activity of the theta waves. The sleep spindle is
electrical activity at a frequency of twelve to fourteen waves per second,
with the same amplitude as theta waves and a shape reminiscent of the
spindle on a loom.

Unlike alpha and theta waves, which appear for minutes at a time,
the K-complex and the sleep spindle are fleeting, lasting between one-
half and a full second. To illustrate the difference between the continuous
alpha and theta waves, which provide the background activity, and the
two short waves, the K-complex and the sleep spindle, let us try to imagine the brain waves as musical notes. The alpha and theta waves are
similar to a monotonic, continuous note played on a violin at a more or
less regular frequency and intensity. These continuous notes are some-

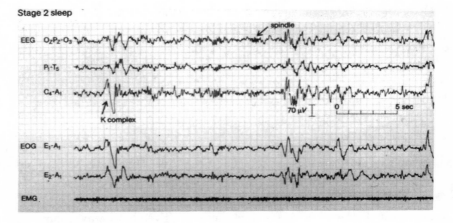

Fig. 6. Sleep stage 2: sleep spindles and K-complexes

times interrupted by shorter notes similar to drumbeats or trumpet notes, representing K-complexes and sleep spindles. The short notes allow us to determine, with a high degree of certainty, that the subject is indeed asleep. In 80 to 100 percent of cases, an attempt to waken the subjects after the appearance of the "sleep notes" will show that they are asleep. The sleep stage characterized by theta background activity and episodic appearances of sleep spindles and K-complexes is known as sleep stage 2.

DELTA WAVES AND DEEP SLEEP

We can therefore decide that a subject is indeed asleep once the transition from stage 1 to stage 2 has taken place. The brain wave recording shows background activity of theta frequency and the episodic appearance of K-complexes and sleep spindles. This, from a subjective standpoint, is still only shallow sleep. In other words, a subject can awaken from stage 2 with relative ease, for although the brain's barriers have been lowered, they have not been lowered completely. Some ten to fifteen minutes after the appearance of K-complexes and sleep spindles, a new type of brain wave—the delta wave—appears. It is slow, of higher voltage than the alpha and theta, and heralds the appearance of deep sleep.

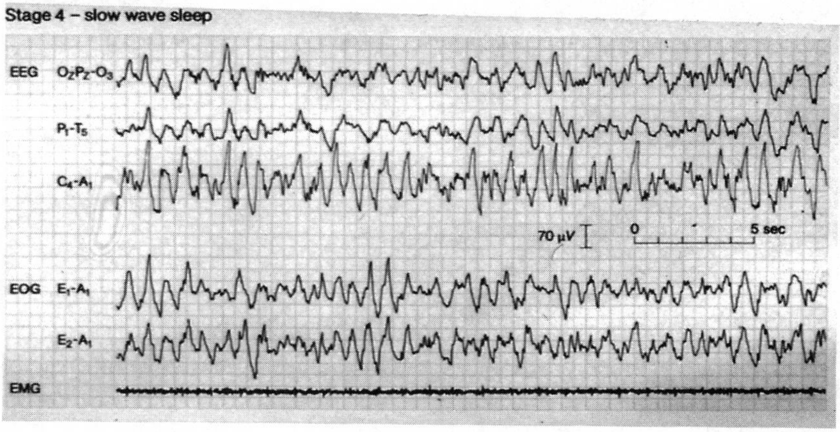

Fig. 7. Sleep stage 4: delta waves

Delta waves show up high and especially prominent against the low background of theta waves, and appear initially on only part of the recording, with theta waves detectable here and there. After a few minutes the theta waves will disappear completely and the recording will display only delta waves. In this stage of sleep, called stage 4, sleep is very deep, muscle relaxation is complete, and heart and breathing rates are slow and regular. In stage 4 it is extremely difficult to detect sleep spindles and K-complexes. The delta waves are so high and so dominant as to obscure any other electrical activity. If sleep is undisturbed, stage 4 will continue for thirty to forty minutes, and only later will the theta waves, sleep spindles, and K-complexes reappear. Then, when it seems that deep sleep has been replaced by shallow sleep, a further change in the electrical activity of the brain will occur. This change remained hidden from researchers for at least twenty years, and when it was discovered by Nathaniel Kleitman and Eugene Aserinsky in 1953, it caused a veritable revolution in the study of sleep.

# 3

# Nathaniel Kleitman

Nathaniel Kleitman is, without doubt, the father of modern sleep research. The story of his life exemplifies every word—written or related—about the fate of the Wandering Jew. He was born in Kishinev, then Russia, in 1895, and at the age of seventeen, after witnessing the pogroms and persecution inflicted upon the Jews, he decided to go to what was then Palestine. At ninety-five years of age, as lucid and ebullient as ever, Kleitman told me that even then he had made up his mind to practice medicine in the Holy Land and had decided to study medicine at the American College in Beirut before settling in Palestine. The outbreak of the First World War cut short his stay in Beirut. As he was a Russian subject and feared the Turks would consider him an enemy alien, he fled to Rhodes. There, as he related somewhat apologetically, he boarded the only ship anchored in the port—which happened to be American—and some weeks later found himself in New York. After completing his master's degree in physiology at Columbia University and spending some time at the University of Georgia, he obtained the post of assistant professor at the University of Chicago, where he established a sleep research laboratory, the first of its kind in the world. In 1939 he published his book *Sleep and Wakefulness,* which rapidly became the Bible of sleep researchers everywhere.

At that time, Kleitman was the only man who made his living solely from the study of sleep, and years later he told me that this obsession did little to advance his academic career. The principal reason behind the lack of interest in sleep was the widely held view that relatively little occurred during sleep and that even if it did, it had absolutely no bearing on the behavior or health of a human being when awake. As we have seen, sleep was viewed as a passive condition which was forced

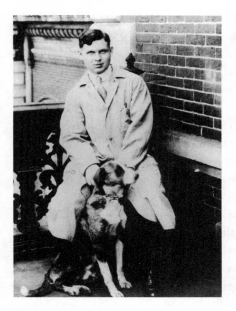

Fig. 8. Nathaniel
Kleitman at the
University of Chi-
cago, about 1925

upon the nervous system as a result of the isolation of the brain from the
other organs of the body. At the beginning of the twentieth century, this
approach was accepted by the majority of the scholars who studied sleep,
including Kleitman himself.

Nathaniel Kleitman was the first scientist to become enchanted by
sleep. His work on the subject dealt with a wide range of subjects, from
breathing during sleep to the sleep characteristics of infants and children,
and his ideas were both original and bold. To prove that the sleep-
wakefulness rhythm is learned, Kleitman and his young assistant spent
a month in total isolation and freezing temperatures in Mammoth Cave
in Kentucky, in order to adapt themselves to sleep-wakefulness rhythms
of twenty-one and twenty-eight hours. Although his assistant succeeded,
Kleitman failed to disengage himself from the twenty-four-hour rhythm.
As he was so much older than his assistant, he assumed that his advanced
age had prevented him from adapting to the conditions of the experiment.

The discovery which truly revolutionized sleep research, that of rapid
eye movement (REM) sleep, was made in 1953, in Kleitman's laboratory,
by a young doctoral student named Eugene Aserinsky. Like many other
scientific discoveries, this was stumbled upon by chance, and there are

several versions of the precise circumstances under which it was made. William Dement, Kleitman's disciple and successor, has provided us with an eyewitness account. Dement began his studies at the University of Chicago Medical School in 1951 and set his sights on specializing in psychiatry. Kleitman's lecture on sleep, which was given as part of a course on neurophysiology, changed his life. He went to see Kleitman and asked for a job in the sleep laboratory. At the time, Aserinsky was studying for his doctorate in physiology with Kleitman. Thus Dement, Aserinsky, and Kleitman formed the first research group in the field of sleep.

Kleitman attached great importance to the slow eye movements which accompany the process of falling asleep. As a great part of the cerebral cortex is committed to controlling eye movements, he theorized that there was a strong connection between the slow eye movements and the depth of sleep. Consequently, he decided to examine whether slow eye movements appeared at any other times during sleep. In the spring of 1951, before Dement had joined the team, he authorized Aserinsky to conduct tests on the subject. To avoid having to spend many sleepless nights, Aserinsky began by observing infants, who also sleep during the day. In his initial observations, Aserinsky immediately saw that the infants' slow eye movements when falling asleep were replaced by rapid eye movements once they had fallen asleep, and that they were identical to eye movements during wakefulness. Once Aserinsky and Kleitman had succeeded in recording rapid eye movements in adults, they were convinced that the cause was either noise or a malfunction in the recording instruments. In order to ascertain that these were indeed true eye movements, Aserinsky asked observers to watch the eyes of the sleeping subjects closely while the recording instruments did their work. He wanted to be completely sure that the eyes did indeed move during sleep and thus eliminate the possibility of a technical fault. It quickly became clear that it was very easy to observe rapid eye movements through the eyelids of the sleeping subject.

It was at this time that Dement asked to join the sleep laboratory staff. He says that had his shyness not prevented him from asking Kleitman to permit him to join the staff earlier, it might easily have been he, not Aserinsky, who made the historic discovery of rapid eye movements during sleep. Dement, too, finds it difficult to determine exactly who discovered that rapid eye movements are connected with dreaming, but he argues that the idea was probably Kleitman's, although it is entirely possible that both Aserinsky and Kleitman came up with it at the same time, each in his own way. Dement's first task in Kleitman's laboratory was to awaken the sleeping subjects when rapid eye movements were detected and ask them whether they had been dreaming. The results were both dramatic and remarkable: in complete contrast to other stages of sleep, when the subjects were awakened from sleep characterized by rapid eye movements, they were able to clearly remember a detailed dream.

In a paper published in the journal *Science* in 1953, which became the cornerstone of modern sleep research, Aserinsky and Kleitman called this type of sleep REM sleep. REM sleep is also known today by several other names—"dream sleep," "paradoxical sleep," and "active sleep"—but for convenience I shall use the term *REM sleep* to describe this type of sleep in humans, and *paradoxical sleep* when referring to animals.

Why was REM sleep not discovered until 1953? On the face of it, everything was in place earlier; the first recordings of brain activity during sleep had been made as early as the 1930s, and the variations in brain waves between the conditions of REM sleep and deep sleep were considerable. The answer to this question is disappointing in its simplicity. When I asked Kleitman why he had not discerned REM sleep earlier, he replied, "Because until 1953 we had not bothered to conduct continuous recordings throughout the night." The immediate reason for this had been economy; to save recording paper, sleep recordings had been made either for only a few minutes every two or three hours, or only during the first hour of sleep. As rapid eye movements only begin to appear some ninety minutes after the subject has fallen asleep, and then only for a period of five to ten minutes, it is very easy to miss them. This is an outstanding example of the great effect that erroneous concepts may have on research methods. It is almost certain that the assumption that sleep was a passive and insignificant condition made a significant contribution to parsimony in research methods.

REM SLEEP

Approximately an hour and a half after falling asleep, the physiological changes which indicate the first appearance of REM sleep occur. The

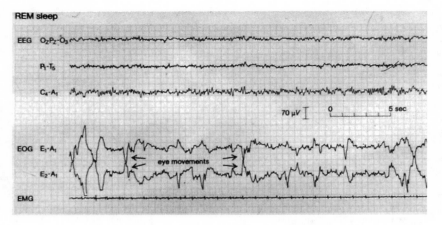

Fig. 9. REM sleep: rapid eye movements are marked by arrows

brain waves show characteristic variations: theta waves—this time without K-complexes or sleep spindles—and short bursts of alpha wave activity which, when appearing during sleep, indicate a high level of alertness. The brain waves in REM sleep are in fact almost completely identical to those in stage 1, which we have defined as half sleep or the transitional stage. We may therefore conclude that REM sleep is shallow and that awakening from it is easy. But that is not the case, for REM sleep is deep, although under special conditions awakening from it can be very easy. The combination of electrical activity in the brain, which indicates shallow sleep, and deep sleep (from a subjective standpoint) has given this type of sleep one of its many names—paradoxical sleep. At the same time, the rapid eye movements which attracted the attention of Aserinsky appeared, thus making the discovery of REM sleep possible.

When I first became a sleep researcher, the great similarity between eye movements in REM sleep and eye movements during wakefulness confounded me. In 1969, when I was studying for my bachelor's degree in psychology at the University of Tel Aviv, we made our first sleep recordings with the objective of identifying REM sleep. To my great good fortune and purely by chance, I was given the opportunity of making a little extra money as a sleep technician, doing the night recordings. With the benefit of hindsight I can now say that it was that opportunity which sealed my fate as a sleep researcher. I should point out that, in his first years at least, the sleep researcher is required to spend many sleepless nights watching over the recording instruments and very often, in the small hours of the night, would willingly change places with the subject who is sound asleep in the examination room.

After a few nights, once we had succeeded in obtaining some clear sleep recordings in which we were able easily to identify each stage of sleep, including the dream stage, we decided to invite the head of the Department of Psychology, Prof. Ron Shoval, to take a look at our impressive achievements. The night he came I arrived late to work, and by the time I went into the instrument room, Shoval and my technician colleagues were all standing by the recording instruments, examining the brain waves and eye movements with great interest. When I looked at the recording sheet, I saw that the eye movements were indeed clear and impressive. With a look of great erudition on my face and barely concealed pride in my voice, I said, "What an impressive example of REM sleep," and went on to praise that extraordinary example of sleep to the skies. Only after a few seconds did I become aware of the sniggers all around me. When I raised my head from the recording sheet and looked through the window into the bedroom, to my astonishment I saw our subject lying on his bed bedecked with electrodes—completely engrossed in the book he was reading. The recording equipment had faithfully charted his eye movements as they jumped from line to line in his book. I have no idea what Professor Shoval thought of the "great erudition" displayed that night, but I can only say in my own defense that there is an almost total similarity between the eye movements of a person who is awake and those of REM sleep, and it is very easy to confuse the two.

## SLEEP PARALYSIS

Eye movements and brain waves are not the only indications of REM sleep. Other changes, no less bizarre, also occur. As I mentioned earlier, the skeletal muscles relax during the falling asleep stage and this relaxation reaches its peak in sleep stage 4, the stage of deepest sleep. There is a further change in muscle tonus during REM sleep: it disappears completely. In this type of sleep we are in fact in a condition of total muscular paralysis, and this, too, is a phenomenon caused by a spontaneous variation in brain activity. Just like the mechanism which inhibits nerve impulses sent from the sensory receptors to the cerebral cortex, there is a reverse inhibitory mechanism, from the brain to the muscles. This prevents the transmission of nerve impulses from the motor cerebral cortex, the areas connected with muscle control, to the spinal column. This inhibition of nerve impulses is done by the transmission of special signals from the area known as the brain stem toward the spinal column, and it is these signals which change the characteristics of nerve cell activity in the spinal column and cause paralysis. Why, then, do we have rapid eye movement? Because the control of the eye muscles is not executed via the spinal column but through special nerve fibers protruding from the brain stem, and these fibers remain unaffected by the paralysis.

Some people appear to be fully aware of this motor paralysis which accompanies REM sleep, and it is by no means a pleasant experience. In these instances, the sleeper awakens to an acute sense of paralysis: he is unable to move his hands or feet, has difficulty in detecting his own respiratory movements, and therefore fears that he might not be breathing or even that he is choking. Only his eyes respond to his commands, as they comb the bedroom in panic, as though pleading for help. Most people describing these "sleep paralysis" events recall a panic-stricken experience. As they try to call for help, they are unable to utter a sound, and the fear of choking is succinctly described as the "fear of death" in its fullest sense. Although in most cases this is a one-time or rare event, in some instances it is a regular phenomenon, sometimes occurring several times a week. When the sleep of people suffering from this disorder is recorded, we find that the paralysis always occurs after waking from REM sleep. We can understand from this that the mechanism which inhibits the nerve signals on their way from the motor cerebral cortex to the spinal column is not removed after the sleeper has awakened, and thus the commands to the muscles continue to be inhibited during wakefulness. Even without outside intervention, an attack of sleep paralysis will subside on its own after a few minutes, but touching the paralyzed subject, or even calling his or her name, will immediately terminate it.

There is another outstanding example of muscle paralysis where people fall asleep as soon as their heads touch the pillow and immediately sink into REM sleep, without passing through any of the first four stages.

These people can enter REM sleep directly while standing, sitting, or even driving a car. The attack causes them to lose control of their muscles, which is potentially extremely dangerous. This disorder is called narcolepsy, and I shall describe it in detail in Chapter 20.

As we scan the history of discoveries in the field of sleep, it seems that we are looking at a huge jigsaw puzzle, where additional pieces regularly fall into place. Many new pieces have been slotted only recently. It became clear, for example, that the great regularity of both the respiratory and pulse rates typifying the stages of deep sleep is replaced by irregularity. In REM sleep, the respiratory and pulse rates undergo radical fluctuations, as though the sleeper were in the throes of a strong emotional upset.

An additional finding was first reported some four years prior to the discovery of REM sleep but fitted into the puzzle of REM sleep only years later. German scientists discovered that the sleep of the male was characterized by a number of nocturnal penile erections which took place every ninety minutes. The researchers thought that these erections were probably a source of dreams, but they knew nothing of REM sleep. It only became clear in the 1960s that an erection indeed accompanies REM sleep.

# The Rhythm of Sleep

The appearance of sleep stages during the night is not a random process but an organized and definitive one. This makes life somewhat easier for the sleep researcher. The sleep sequence can best be described with the aid of a hypnogram of the sleep recording. As there are considerable variations in the sleep sequence and organization of sleep stages at various ages, I shall first describe the sleep sequence of a typical young man in his twenties.

Let us set out on our nocturnal journey at the moment the light is switched off. As soon as his eyes are closed and the preparations for sleep get under way, alpha waves indicating relaxation appear, and a few minutes later our subject will pass from restful wakefulness to sleep stage 1. If he suffers no undue sleep disturbances, then two to five minutes later, after we have discerned sleep spindles and K-complexes against the even background of the theta waves, he will move into sleep stage 2. Early in the night, this stage will also swiftly pass, and after some ten minutes we should be able to see the first incursion of the high, slow delta waves on the recording sheet. While the delta waves still account for less than 50 percent of the recording, this is sleep stage 3, an interim stage between the shallow sleep of stage 2 and the deep sleep of stage 4. As in stage 1, the transition between wakefulness and sleep, stage 3 is of brief duration. When stage 4 appears, in no time at all the only waves we can see on the recording are delta waves. Now follows a certain stabilization of the electrical activity, and for the following thirty or forty minutes there will be no change in the brain waves, no gross movements of the trunk or limbs, and it will be very difficult to awaken the subject. This is usually the time when the researcher can leave his post for a few moments and enjoy a cup of coffee.

A body movement or several gross body movements are the first indication that a change is about to occur in the sleep sequence. The
sleeper changes position, turns from side to side, or turns over from his
back to his stomach. Stage 4 has been interrupted. These gross body
movements usually cause erratic recordings, which then subside to show
that the subject has returned not to a deep sleep but to a shallower sleep
stage—stage 3 or even 2. Further body movements will appear some five
or six minutes later, heralding exactly what the sleep researcher has
expectantly been awaiting—the appearance of REM sleep. The sleep
spindles and K-complexes will suddenly disappear, as will the muscle
tonus. The eye movement recording track will begin a frantic "dance"
and the eyes themselves will jump from side to side for several minutes.
The duration of the first dream period is usually short—no more than
five to ten minutes—and, like stage 4, it concludes with gross body movements. Their appearance at the end of certain sleep stages acts something
like a punctuation mark—or, more precisely, exclamation mark—which
the brain has inserted into this particular "sentence."

The body movements bring about a change in the sleep stage; REM
sleep is over and stage 1, the transitional stage, will reappear for a minute
or two, followed immediately by stage 2, the shallow sleep stage, and
another sleep cycle has begun. The sleeper will again pass through stages
2, 3, and 4, at the conclusion of which REM sleep will again appear.
There are, however, several differences between the first and second
sleep cycles, and they will also be discerned in subsequent cycles. The
duration of deep sleep in stages 3 and 4 decreases because the duration
of shallow sleep in stage 2 increases, and the duration of the second REM
sleep is longer than that of the first. Instead of lasting five to seven
minutes, it will last twelve to fifteen. Apart from the variations in the
relative duration of the sleep stages, the second cycle will not contain
changes in either brain wave characteristics or the appearance of gross
body movements. The first sleep cycle, which is measured from the moment of falling asleep to the appearance of the first REM period, is also
called "REM latency" and lasts for approximately an hour and a half.
The following sleep cycles, which are measured from the beginning of
one period of REM sleep to the beginning of the next, also last for about
ninety minutes. This is of great interest because in certain types of sleep

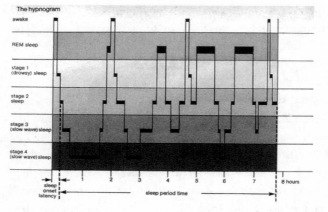

Fig. 10. Hypnogram of a young adult

disorders REM latency is shortened, and this helps in the diagnosis of the disorder.

The third sleep cycle, which begins once the second REM period is over, comprises still less deep sleep, and a longer period of light sleep. The third REM period is relatively long—about twenty to twenty-five minutes—while the fourth sleep cycle contains an even smaller amount of deep sleep, with the lion's share being stage 2 sleep. The duration of the fourth REM sleep is about the same as the third, up to twenty minutes or perhaps a little longer. As the sleep cycles last for some ninety minutes, their number per night depends on the duration of sleep; a young person's sleep is usually composed of four or five such cycles, while an older person has fewer.

## SLEEP FROM INFANCY TO OLD AGE

Experience has taught us that sleep varies with age. While infants spend a great deal of time sleeping, the elderly usually suffer from interrupted sleep and consequently doze off many times during the day. So how does the rhythm of sleep vary with age?

One of the most unexpected findings which awaited the sleep researchers in the laboratory concerned the sleep of infants. When adults say they have "slept like a baby," we automatically assume their sleep was particularly tranquil. But is the sleep of infants really all that peaceful?

Meticulous observation of a sleeping baby, especially during the first days of his or her life, will reveal that the infant enjoys two completely different types of sleep, one of which was first observed by Aserinsky and Kleitman in 1953. While this sleep is accompanied by rapid eye movements, their appearance does not signal the onset of complete motor paralysis as it does with adults. The baby in this type of sleep is in a state of increased motoric activity. It is subject not to gross body movements but rather to small, often spasmodic movements of the fingers and toes, hands and feet, and facial muscles. From time to time, the movements include those facial expressions associated with crying, anger, and rejection. Moreover, the first smile in the life of the human infant appears during REM sleep, and this is why REM sleep in infants is also called "active sleep." In this sleep stage in infants, the majority of brain waves are theta waves just like those of the adult during REM sleep. The second type of sleep is indeed quiet and peaceful, with no gross or small body movements—in fact, exactly as we define "baby sleep." Developed delta waves and sleep spindles cannot be discerned during the infant's sleep in the first days or weeks of life: electrical brain activity is irregular and disorganized.

What do these two types of infants' sleep tell us? Not unexpectedly, infants' active sleep is indeed analogous to adults' REM sleep. The brain's inhibitory mechanisms which block the transmission of nerve impulses to the skeletal muscles are still immature, and this results in increased small body movements. However, these mechanisms will mature during the first year of life, and the agitated body movements evident during REM sleep will disappear at the same time, leaving only the rapid eye movements. Sleep stages 2, 3, and 4 will develop from this "nonactive" peaceful sleep.

Yet it was not only the REM sleep that surprised the researchers but also its relative duration. In the first weeks of its life, the infant spends about half of its sleeping time in active sleep, and this will decrease gradually during the first year, stabilizing at about 25–30 percent at one year of age. The infant's sleep rhythm is also faster than that of the adult. The time which elapses between one active sleep and the next is only some sixty minutes, unlike the ninety-minute REM cycle of the adult.

When does the brain "clock" that controls active sleep start to tick? There are those who, based on their observations of motoric movements of fetuses, claim that active sleep can be discerned even before birth, from the sixth month of pregnancy onward, and this claim has been substantiated by a study conducted in the Technion Sleep Laboratory. The study included the continuous recording of fetal movements over a period of several hours, in women in their sixth and seventh months of pregnancy. We found that the movements of the fetus varied cyclically, with the intervals between the peaks of fetal activity standing at some sixty minutes, which is identical to the interval between two consecutive periods of active sleep during the first days following the infant's birth. These findings pose numerous questions: Why does the infant spend so much time in active sleep? Is this type of sleep especially important during infancy? Is it more important than quiet sleep? In Chapter 12, in my discussion of the possible roles played by REM sleep, I will try to answer these puzzling questions.

An adult's sleep rhythm is consolidated approximately between his or her tenth and twentieth year, and the sleep stages are then divided into approximately 20–25 percent REM sleep, 20–25 percent deep sleep as in stages 3 and 4, and the remainder in stage 2 shallow sleep. "Bedtime" also includes a certain percentage of transitional sleep and wakefulness, which are usually linked to the body movements that punctuate the transitional period between sleep stages.

Human aging is bound up with substantial changes in the quality of sleep. Most elderly people complain a great deal about frequent interruptions of their night's sleep, early-morning awakenings, and a tendency to doze during the day. All of these complaints have a sound physiological basis. Electrophysiological sleep recordings in elderly people show characteristic variations which explain the subjective complaints. The most pronounced finding in the sleep structure of elderly persons is a decrease in the duration of deep sleep. While the duration of deep sleep in young persons in their thirties varies between 20 and 25 percent of their sleep, that of elderly persons in their seventies or eighties is only 5 to 10 percent. Because of this considerable decrease in the duration of deep sleep, elderly persons' sleep is mainly comprised of REM sleep, which remains about 10–20 percent of their total sleep, and stage 2 shallow sleep. More important than the changes in the composition of sleep stage is the change in sleep consolidation of elderly people. As I shall discuss later on, in-

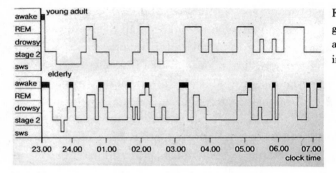

Fig. 11. Hypnograms for a young adult and an elderly individual

creased awakenings from sleep frequently signal aging, much as wrinkles and graying hair.

## SLEEP TO GROW

For hundreds of years people believed that, like the other characteristics of the human race, sickness and health were dependent upon mysterious fluids which flowed through the body, and therefore they ascribed the principal cause of sickness to an imbalance of these fluids. Likewise, the relative quantity of each fluid present in the body was supposed to determine a person's personality, and to this very day we use the adjective "phlegmatic" to describe someone who is apathetic, slow, and tedious. The term is, of course, derived from the word *phlegm,* which was one of the four principal bodily fluids in ancient Greek medicine.

Neither Hippocrates nor Galen, the fathers of the fluid theory, had any idea of the existence of hormones, those products of internal secretions carried in the bloodstream. The twentieth-century development of endocrinology, which deals with the study of hormones and their effects, revived the ancient concept of the importance of bodily fluids and their significant effects on health and sickness. It is therefore hardly surprising that the discovery of the variations in nervous system activity during the transition from wakefulness to sleep posed the following question to many researchers: Do changes occur in hormonal secretion at the same time? As with the nervous system, the hormones secreted by glands located throughout the body play their part in coordination and control of numerous physiological systems. There are those, like sex hormones, which affect the function of many specific organs, and also general systems including the brain. Some affect the functioning of all the bodily systems and determine metabolic and growth rate of the organs.

The secretion of the growth hormone was the first one to be studied in the field of sleep. The discovery that the growth hormone is secreted by the pituitary gland was made in 1945, and the hormone's important role in the growth of soft tissues and bones became known soon afterward. It was then believed to be secreted during the day after meals, during physical exertion, and under conditions of mental stress. Therefore in 1968, when Takahashi and his colleagues reported that the daily secretion of the hormone reaches its peak in both children and adults immediately after falling asleep, during the deep sleep of stages 3 and 4, the surprise was tremendous. In order to examine the possible causal connection between growth hormone secretion and sleep mechanisms, hormone secretion was investigated following changes in sleeping habits. When sleep was delayed by twelve hours, the peak of hormone secretion indeed was delayed accordingly. When sleep was disturbed more than two or three hours, an additional secretion peak appeared after sleep had been resumed. Hence we may conclude that the process of falling asleep and entering the deep sleep stages 3 and 4 causes the secretion of growth hormone by the pituitary gland.

Other studies have shown that the secretion of the growth hormone is unrelated to the process of falling asleep but is related to the appearance of the high, slow delta waves which indicate deep sleep. Yet there is evidence that the mechanism responsible for the secretion of the hormone during sleep is not identical with the one responsible for deep sleep, and the two phenomena can be separated by administering medication. Growth hormone secretion can be completely suppressed without affecting the normal course of deep sleep and, at the same time, the appearance of deep sleep can be prevented without affecting the secretion of the hormone. We may therefore assume the existence of two separate mechanisms which are closely linked.

The secretion of other hormones does not correspond as closely as that of the growth hormone to the rhythm of the sleep stages. Cortisol, for example, is a hormone secreted by the adrenal gland which affects metabolic rate. It is vigorously secreted under conditions of stress, and one of its primary functions is the mobilization of energy in emergency

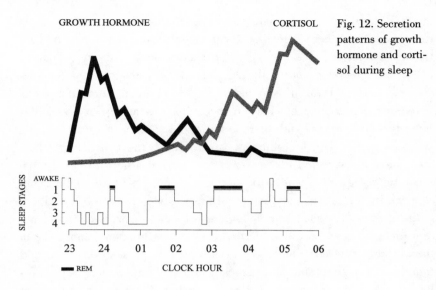

GROWTH HORMONE          CORTISOL

Fig. 12. Secretion patterns of growth hormone and cortisol during sleep

SLEEP STAGES

AWAKE
1
2
3
4

23   24   01   02   03   04   05   06

■ REM          CLOCK HOUR

conditions. It is therefore hardly surprising that the awakening process is accompanied by increased cortisol secretion in order to "prepare" the organism to combat the physical demands of wakefulness. The rise in cortisol secretion begins in the middle of the sleep period and increases gradually with a series of pulses, until it reaches its peak at awakening. The difference between the cortisol level in the blood while falling asleep, and that at awakening, is so great that the interpretation of cortisol blood levels is meaningless without knowing exactly when the sample was taken.

As the secretion of cortisol is not continuous but comprised of gradually increasing peaks, there are those who argue that REM sleep, which appears mainly in the second part of sleep, is the factor responsible for increased secretion of the hormone. There is, however, no immediate change in cortisol secretion when sleep is put off by a few hours, for that requires several days. This means that, in contrast to the growth hormone, cortisol secretion is controlled by an independent biological clock which is not usually closely coordinated with the sleep clock.

There are, however, other hormones whose secretion is coordinated with sleep, especially during critical periods of life. The gonadotropic hormones, for example, which are also secreted by the pituitary gland, are responsible for the regulation of the secretion of sex hormones from the gonads, and thereby for the development of the sex organs and for the appearance of the secondary sex characteristics at puberty. At puberty, they are secreted mainly during sleep. Measurement of the gonadotropic hormones' level prior to and at the end of puberty does not reveal variations in hormone level when the subject is asleep or awake. At puberty, on the other hand, there is increased hormone secretion during sleep compared with wakefulness. Like cortisol, the gonadotropic hormones are not secreted continuously but are pulsatile; in other words, the pituitary gland releases the hormones into the bloodstream every ninety minutes. It was later found that this method of secretion is critical to the effects of the gonadotropic hormones on the sex organs. It appeared that the sex organs were unable to "decode" the hormonal signals from the pituitary unless the hormones are secreted in pulses every hour and a half. A permanent and continuous secretion of the gonadotropic hormones has an inhibitory rather than stimulatory effect on the function of the gonads.

Thus, it appears that sleep plays an important role in regulating hormonal secretions. During sleep, the endocrine organs come to life and secrete into the bloodstream hormones that affect the entire body.

# The Twenty-five Hour Day

Having examined the rhythm of sleep stages in all its complexity, we can now move on to the rhythm of sleep and wakefulness. Although adults tend to take the regularity of our sleep habits for granted, this is not the case in our early years. While the birth of a new baby in a family is bound up with feelings of joy and fulfillment, it is also accompanied by an extended period of change in the sleep habits of the happy parents. They are obliged to forgo their customary uninterrupted night's sleep and wake up every few hours to attend to the needs of the new arrival. The infant's sleep habits are an inseparable part of conversations heard in the waiting rooms of doctors and child-care clinics. There we can find parents who are totally exhausted, especially those who have recently celebrated the birth of their first child, and who have given up hope of their child ever adapting to normal sleep habits. They call grandparents to the rescue and decamp for the nearest hotel for one or two nights' sleep in order to recharge their depleted batteries. But sooner or later nearly every baby adapts itself to its parents' desires: sleeping during the night and staying awake during the day. In most babies, this process of adaptation to the outside world is gradual and takes place during the first six months of life. In the first month, the baby wakes and sleeps every four hours, and some parents and pediatricians recommend planning this rhythm by feeding the baby every four hours, which is the "natural" sleep rhythm. But the number of nocturnal awakenings gradually decreases from two or three per night to one or two, and the number of daytime sleeping periods decreases at the same time. At approximately six months, much to the relief of the parents, the baby begins sleeping almost through the night and the sleep-wakefulness rhythm stabilizes at twenty-four hours.

Does the infant acquire sleep-wakefulness habits from its environment, or is the sleep-wakefulness rhythm also controlled by an internal
"biological clock"? One of the first researchers to study this question was
Nathaniel Kleitman, who believed that the sleep-wakefulness rhythm is
learned. In order to investigate the development of the rhythm in infants,
Kleitman traced the sleep of infants who determined when to sleep of
their own volition. He allowed them to sleep and awaken naturally, and
to be fed when they indicated by crying or restlessness that they were
hungry. Kleitman's book *Sleep and Wakefulness,* first published in 1939
and reissued in 1963, summarized everything that was then known about
sleep, referring to more than four thousand scientific sources. The jacket
of the second edition faithfully depicts the formulation of the twenty-four-
hour sleep rhythm of one of Kleitman's subjects. As we can see in the
illustration, the night sleep periods lengthen while the daytime sleep
periods become shorter from the fourth month of the infant's life. But
those of us blessed with sharp vision can detect something else; diagonal
configurations which indicate the permanent shifting of waking times
from one day to the next. If the infant woke and was fed at 2 P.M. on one
day, the next day it awoke at 2:15 P.M., at 2:30 P.M. the next day, and so
on. These diagonal configurations can be further emphasized by doubling
the recording sheet. Kleitman himself was aware of them and attributed
them to the lunar cycle.

For many years after the publication of his book, these "Milky Ways"
did not gain the attention of sleep researchers. It was only after the
characteristics of the biological clock which controls sleep-wakefulness
became clear that the phenomenon was explained. During the first months
of life, sleep and wakefulness are controlled by the biological clock, the
periodicity of which is not an integer of 24 hours—in other words, the
cycle's duration is not 3, 4, or 6 hours. If that were the case, then daily
sleeping and waking times would be identical from day to day. If, for
example, the infant has a cycle of 3.5 hours and on a certain day wakes
up at 7 A.M., the infant will awaken at 7:30 A.M. the next day, at 8 A.M.
the day after, and so on. Likewise, there will be drifting into and out of
sleep for about half an hour at all the other waking and sleeping times,
and this will show up on the recording as diagonal lines.

Bernie Webb and I conducted a study similar to Kleitman's. We
traced the consolidation of sleep-wakefulness rhythm in a large group of

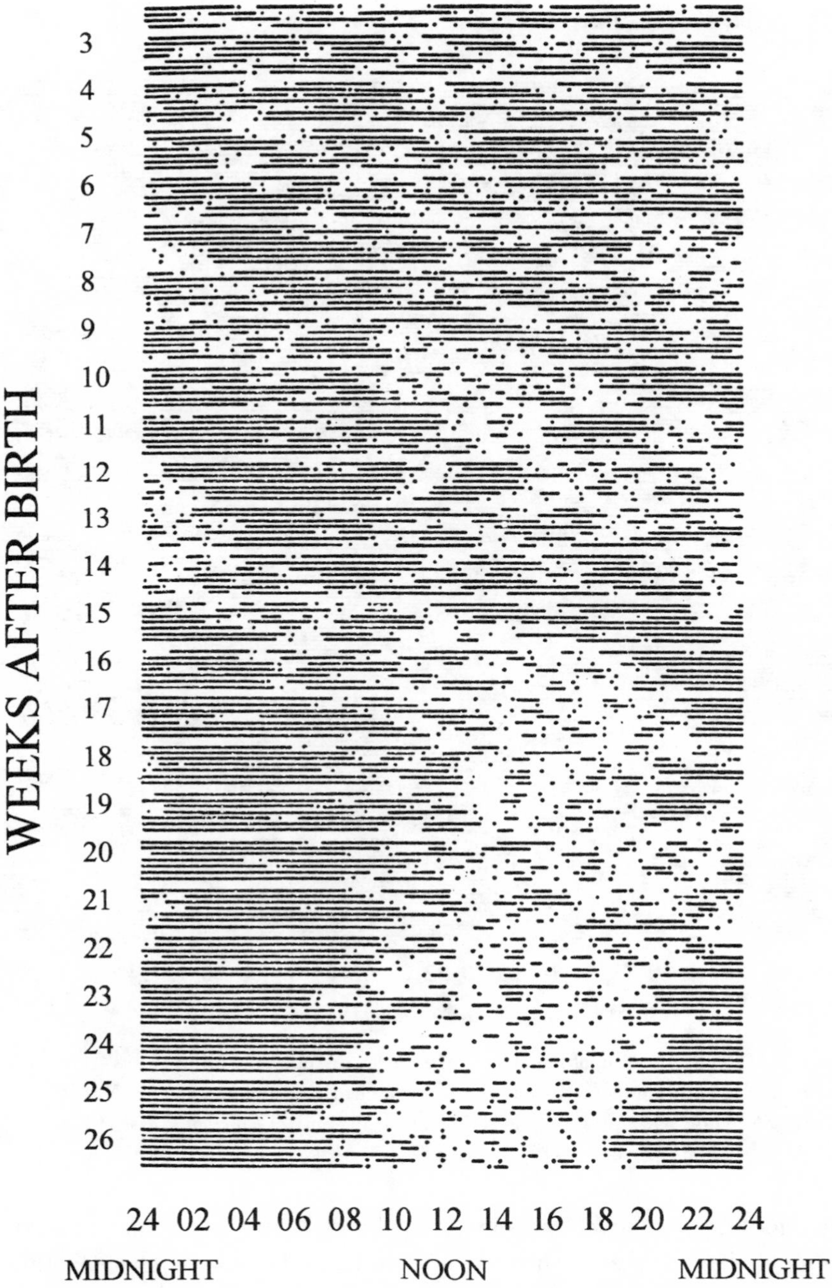

Fig. 13. Consolidation of sleep-wakefulness rhythm in an infant: black lines indicate sleep, dots indicate feeding, and white patches indicate wakefulness. From the jacket of N. Kleitman's *Sleep and Wakefulness*, 2d ed. (Chicago: University of Chicago Press, 1963).

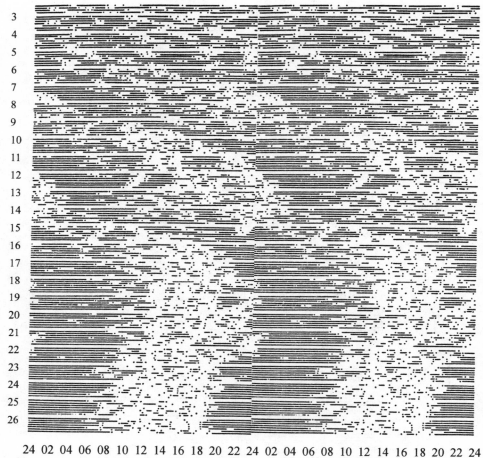

Fig. 14. Doubled plotting of the sleep-wakefulness rhythm: the "Milky Ways" that indicate the daily shift of sleep periods can be seen clearly. From the jacket of N. Kleitman's *Sleep and Wakefulness*, 2d ed. (Chicago: University of Chicago Press, 1963).

infants who were given the same freedom as Kleitman's babies to wake
up and sleep as they wished. At first we had great doubts about finding
mothers who would volunteer to participate in the experiment, but they
were rapidly dispelled. As it turned out, many mothers volunteered and
cooperated enthusiastically; some even said that the freedom of sleep and

wakefulness given to their babies made their own lives a great deal easier. The mothers kept a precise record of all the babies' sleep periods and feeding times over a period of at least two months, and upon analyzing the records we found that the sleep-wakefulness rhythm was very similar to that on the jacket of Kleitman's book. None of the babies who participated in the study had a 4-hour rhythm but one that was either slightly shorter or longer—3.5 or 4.5 hours. Some of the mothers even noted this and succeeded in planning their daily schedule according to their babies' projected sleeping and feeding times.

Two major changes occur in the sleep-wakefulness rhythm during the first year of the infant's life. A single and continuous sleep period and a period of continuous wakefulness begin to emerge, and at the same time a pattern of coordination between the sleep-wakefulness rhythm and the demands of the external environment slowly begins to develop. The rate of change varies from baby to baby. In our study, we found great differences in the age at which the fast rhythm was replaced by the sleep-wakefulness rhythm of the adult. Some babies adapted themselves to habits dictated by the environment within two to three months, while others did not manage to do so even after a year. Our experience in the treatment of sleep disorders in infants has shown that a small number of babies do not adapt even at two or three years of age. We shall see what can be done about these obstinate young people later.

What, then, is the reason behind the infant's sleep-wakefulness rhythm, a rhythm which is not an integer of 24 hours? Could the adults' "sleep clock" also not be a 24-hour clock? The characteristics of this sleep clock must be examined in total isolation from all the environmental factors which regulate our time. We are exposed to innumerable stimuli during a 24-hour period. The urgent ringing of the alarm clock wakes us up in the morning knowing that if we do not get out of bed in time, we shall be late for work or school. The school bell or the factory horn heralds the start of the day, meal times, coffee breaks, and recesses, as well as the end of the day. Many people who fall asleep in front of the television set describe this falling asleep as a reflex response conditional to a range of stimuli which are linked to the body's sitting position and the familiar notes of the evening newscast's signature tune. There are those who attest that they wake up in the morning "exactly one minute before the alarm clock rings," a habit formed over many years.

As we can learn to increase brain wave activity with the help of biofeedback, it is not surprising that we can learn to fall asleep and wake up at set times. But are our sleeping habits formed only by learning and conditioning? If they are, then why is it so difficult for us to adapt to new sleeping habits, as when we fly through several time zones or have to work during the night and sleep during the day? The only way to investigate the origin of the sleep-wakefulness rhythm is to isolate subjects from the outside world and examine how they organize their sleeping and waking time. In a "time-free" environment, as it is called in research literature, subjects decide for themselves when to go to sleep and for how long, and when to wake up. For a limited time they enjoy complete freedom; no longer subject to the tyranny of alarm clocks, diaries, and schedules, they become "masters of time." They decide when to switch on the lights and create day, and when to switch them off and create night.

## SLEEP IN A TIME-FREE ENVIRONMENT

The first studies on the effects of the removal of "time cues" on the sleep-wakefulness rhythm were conducted by isolating the subjects in deep caverns. There it was possible completely to remove the effects of alternating light and darkness, the accompanying variations in temperature and humidity, and the wide range of social stimuli to which the human being is exposed during each twenty-four-hour day. For the first time, the study of the subjects' sleep was done through reporting in diaries the times of going to bed and waking up, as well as daily changes in body temperature, blood pressure, and pulse rate. The subjects were isolated for periods varying from weeks to months, during which they were given no information about whether it was night or day outside the cavern.

Although it might be assumed that the sleep-wakefulness rhythm in isolation would be different from that in a natural environment, the change in sleeping habits was extremely surprising. The sleep-wakefulness rhythm of the isolated subjects was maintained, but the duration of its cycle—the interval between one sleeping time and the next—was invariably longer than twenty-four hours, and this lengthened cycle varied from one subject to the next. In some the cycle lengthened to twenty-five hours, while others adopted a twenty-seven- or twenty-eight-

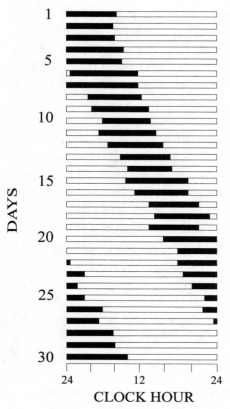

Fig. 15. Sleep-wakefulness rhythm in a "time-free" environment: dark bars indicate periods of sleep

**CLOCK HOUR**

hour cycle, or even longer. As the sun rises approximately every twenty-four hours, a person who has a twenty-seven-hour cycle will delay his sleeping time by three hours every geophysical day. So if, on the first day of his isolation, he decides to go to sleep at midnight, he will do so at 3 A.M. the next day, at 6 A.M. the day after that, and at 9 A.M. the third day. After eight sleep-wakefulness cycles, he will return to his starting point and once again go to sleep at midnight. This variation in sleeping and waking times is similar to that observed in babies who determined their feeding and sleeping times by themselves. The rhythm, which is not dependent on the external environment and which deviates from the twenty-four-hour rhythm, is called the "circadian rhythm" (from Latin *circa*, meaning "about," and *dies*, "day")—that is, a rhythm of about one day.

Can this phenomenon typify a small group of people who are not representative of the entire population? This was one of the first questions which arose concerning the lengthening of the sleep-wakefulness rhythm in isolation. People who agree to be isolated for weeks and months of their own free will are probably no ordinary individuals, so the first experiments comprised only a few subjects, some of whom had already participated in many studies. The most famous of these was Michel Siffre, a French speleologist who spent some time at a depth of nearly one hundred feet below the earth's surface in the Midnight Cave in Texas. With electrodes connected to his body to record the physiological parameters required to determine the mode of his sleep, he entered the cave on February 14 and remained there for one hundred consecutive days. His sleep-wakefulness rhythm lengthened to twenty-six hours, although the periodicity of the cycle varied during his isolation, sometimes drastically, to days as long as thirty and thirty-two hours. Siffre has documented his experiences during long periods of isolation in his book *Beyond Time.*

Many additional findings have accumulated over recent years which substantiate the assumption that the lengthening of the sleep-wakefulness rhythm exists in humans and is an expression of the basic property of the biological clock which controls sleep and wakefulness. Since the 1970s, scores if not hundreds of people have been isolated in time-free environments with identical results: almost immediately after the first day of isolation from the environment, their sleep-wakefulness rhythm lengthened to more than twenty-four hours.

Many of the studies on sleep-wakefulness rhythms in a time-free environment were conducted in a small, picturesque German town called Erling-Andachs, which, incidentally, is also famed for its brewery. There, German physiologist Jürgen Aschoff established an institute for the study of "biological clocks" which was, until its closure at the end of the 1980s, the destination of pilgrimages made by sleep researchers from all over the world. Aschoff, too, began his research of biological rhythms purely by chance. As a student, he studied the mechanisms of human resistance to cold, and as his experiments became more prolonged, he began to observe more closely the daily changes in body temperature that were unrelated to the conditions of the experiment. Seeking to understand these spontaneous variations in body temperature, he methodically stud-

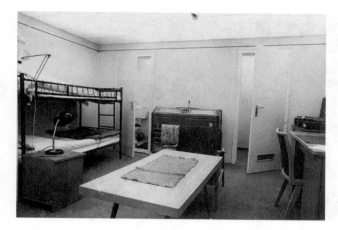

Fig. 16. The bun-
ker at Ehrling-
Andachs, Germany,
in which studies on
sleep in a time-free
environment were
conducted

ied all his physiology literature but was unable to find a reasonable explanation. In the books which devoted a few lines to periodic changes in
body temperature, he discovered that there was some contention between
those who claimed that the source of this rhythm was internal and those
who argued that it was external. After reading all he could find about
biological "clocks," he concluded that there could only be one verification of the existence of an internal rhythm which was not dependent upon
the external environment. If, under constant conditions, the rhythm did
not change even if the periodicity of the cycle might deviate from twenty-
four hours, there could be no doubt that the external environment had
no effect on the biological clock. This assumption led him to try isolating
animals from alternating environmental light and darkness in order to
study their activity-rest rhythm.

Aschoff and his colleagues first experimented with isolating humans
in 1962. This was followed by more than two hundred similar experiments
conducted at the institute in subterranean living quarters custom-built
for this purpose. These small apartments were fully equipped for long
stays under conditions of total isolation from the external environment:
one of them was even isolated from the earth's magnetic field. Each apartment could house groups of subjects in isolation in order to examine the
mutual influence between humans on sleep-wakefulness rhythms. Only
7 of the 232 subjects who participated in the Erling-Andachs studies
asked to end the experiment before it had reached its conclusion, and of

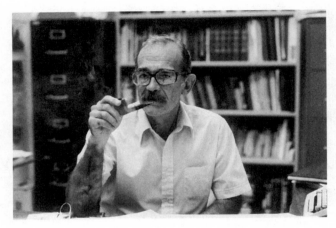

Fig. 17. Bernie
Webb

those, only 3 asked to stop because they were unable to stand the pressure
of isolation. At the end of the isolation period, many of the subjects asked
to participate in further studies, a sure indication that the time spent in
isolation had caused them no harm.

During my sleep research studies at the University of Florida, I participated in one of the first studies conducted in the United States on the
sleep-wakefulness rhythm in isolation. The year I joined Bernie Webb's
staff as a research assistant, he was studying sleep rhythm in a time-free
environment. Unlike the experiments in which the research staff kept
track of their subjects by means of under-floor sensors or sleep diaries,
the Florida study used continuous recording of brain waves, eye movements, and muscle tonus throughout the isolation period. As few caves
are to be found in the state of Florida, subjects remained in completely
soundproof rooms which were totally isolated from the external environment. Each room contained a kitchen corner, a chemical toilet, and a
washbasin. The subjects communicated with the experimenters super-
vising the recording instruments in the control room by means of notes
passed out of the cell. They ordered breakfast, lunch, or dinner whenever
they felt hungry, and a restaurant close to the campus was on "twenty-
four-hour alert" to supply meals at any time of the day or night.

I recall that in the planning stage I expressed grave doubts regarding
the response of potential subjects for a stay of "at least one month" in a
cell-like room no bigger than some fourteen square feet. But much to my

surprise, once the experiment and its conditions were announced in the campus bulletin, the telephone in the laboratory did not stop ringing. The experiment, which was planned for twelve subjects, attracted scores of student volunteers who stood in line outside the laboratory and tried to persuade Professor Webb to accept them. Screening and interviewing revealed that all the candidates were completely normal, not a group of bizarre recluses. As expected, after one or two sleep periods, every one of the subjects switched to a sleep-wakefulness rhythm longer than twenty-four hours.

A further question examined in the study was whether the lengthening of the sleep-wakefulness rhythm in isolation was the result of a change in the subjects' energy balance. As the isolation room offered no possibility of vigorous exercise, there was a big drop in the subjects' physical activity, and this may have affected their sleep "clocks." Half of the subjects were therefore required to engage in strenuous physical activity on exercycles so that their daily expended energy would be similar to that of an average day's work. Their sleep-wakefulness rhythm was not significantly different from that of the subjects who were not required to perform any planned physical activities. The rhythm was lengthened to the same extent in both groups, invalidating the energy explanation.

My own part in the research program focused on another phenomenon which bothered many researchers: the change which occurred in the isolated subjects' sense of time. In all studies where subjects were isolated in a time-free environment, the subjects greatly underestimated the duration of their participation. When they emerged from a month's isolation, they were invariably convinced that only three weeks had elapsed since the beginning of the experiment. As long as the periodicity of the sleep-wakefulness cycle lengthened, the time "lost" in isolation continued to increase. My job was to conduct a controlled examination of the isolated subjects' sense of time. Every few hours, the subjects were asked to send out notes with their estimations of the day of the week and the time of day. They were also asked to estimate the time of day when they switched off the light to go to bed and when they switched it back on upon waking. Every day they were asked to estimate periods of time of less than a few minutes. To avoid giving the subjects any kind of regular cue with which they could estimate time, these tasks were given at varying intervals.

Analysis of the results showed that the subjects were completely unaware of any change in their sleep-wakefulness rhythm. Subjects who switched off the light in the early hours of the morning or during the day in order to sleep, estimated the time at "about midnight," the time that they were accustomed to going to bed in their natural environment. When they woke up, at any hour of the day or night, they estimated the time as "about 7 A.M.," their usual time to rise. However, when they were asked to estimate very short periods of time, no change in their ability to do so was evident. Why, then, were their estimations of time spent in isolation so erroneous? The answer lay in their reliance on earlier sleeping habits when estimating the time of day. When a subject decided to go to bed at 6 A.M. and was convinced that the time was midnight, he erred by six hours, and this error was compounded as the period of isolation continued and as the sleep-wakefulness rhythm lengthened. Therefore, subjects with cycle durations of twenty-seven to twenty-eight hours who spent about a month in isolation lost about a week, because they were unaware of the change which had occurred in their sleeping habits.

The conclusion of the numerous studies in time-free environments is that the source of the sleep-wakefulness rhythm is the nervous system: it is not learned and remains unaffected by the external environment. As the "biological" day is so different from the "geophysical" day, the two clocks, the "body clock" and the "sun clock," must be synchronized.


## SLOW CLOCKS AND FAST CLOCKS

There has to be a coordinating mechanism between the external environment and the biological clock which controls sleep and wakefulness, and it must be flexible enough to allow for deviation from routine. People who work at night and sleep during the day reverse their timetable over a period of several days. A similar thing happens to those who fly through several time zones on their way from continent to continent. The mechanism must indeed be efficient because the "body" and "sun" clocks have to be coordinated each day, and any disruption can seriously disturb the sleep-wakefulness rhythm. The disruption of the coordinating mechanism between someone's sleep-wakefulness clock and environmental rhythms results in his sleep clock behaving in its natural surroundings as though he were isolated in a deep cave. This disruption will have a significant effect on his life, as can be seen by the following striking example.

In 1981 the dean of students at the Technion referred to the Sleep Laboratory a student who was about to be expelled. The reason given for this drastic step was "consistent absence from lectures and examinations due to his inability to wake up in the morning." On interviewing the student, I discovered that although his main problem lay in difficulty in waking up, he also suffered from extreme irregularity in his sleeping habits. He told me that there were days when he went to bed in the evening, just like everyone else, and woke up next morning in time for his first lecture. But there were also nights when he was unable to fall asleep at all and consequently fell asleep during lectures. When he fell asleep in the mornings, he slept through consecutive lectures without even being aware of how many lecturers had taken their place at the front of the class. He added that there was no regularity in his sleeping habits and that when he fell asleep during the day, it was not simply a case of dozing off but a long and continuous sleep which would sometimes go on for hours. After laboratory tests showed that his sleep was normal, we asked him to keep a daily record of his sleep-wakefulness rhythm. The reason behind his sleep disorder became clear after the first ten days: we found that his sleep-wakefulness rhythm behaved as though he were isolated from environmental time cues.

Day by day the student would "delay" his sleeping and waking times by three or four hours. Although the day-to-day changes were less regular than those observed in isolation experiments, it was a simple matter to identify the diagonal configurations which characterized subjects in isolation. The disturbance in his sleep-wakefulness rhythm was the explanation for his complaint. On days in which his sleep-wakefulness rhythm was coordinated with his environment, he managed to fall asleep in the evening just like anyone else, but after a few days, once his sleep had shifted to the daytime hours and coordination was lost, he fell asleep compulsively during lectures and was unable to wake up. Once we had diagnosed the disorder in his sleep timing, we recommended that the dean allow the student to maintain a personal schedule of lectures and examinations which would be determined by his peculiar "sleep clock." As a result, he managed successfully to complete his studies at the Technion.

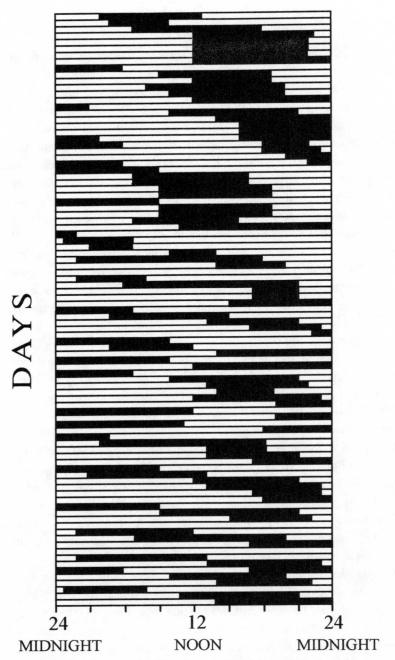

24                    12                    24
MIDNIGHT          NOON          MIDNIGHT

Fig. 18. Sleep-wakefulness rhythm of a patient, showing a lack of coordination between his biological clock and the sun's day: dark bars indicate
periods of sleep

With the help of the student's "sleep diary," we kept track of his sleep-wakefulness rhythm for four full years, thus learning that the functioning of his sleep-wakefulness clock was extremely erratic. There were periods during which the cycle periodicity was twenty-six hours (and thus his daily sleep delay was only two hours), but there were also periods in which periodicity jumped to twenty-nine hours—with a daily delay of five whole hours! Owing to frequent changes in his sleep rhythm duration, he was unable not only to maintain regular sleeping hours but also to maintain a fixed daily schedule. After four years we decided to determine whether any regularity at all existed in what had first appeared to be total chaos. Using computerized statistical analyses, we examined in detail those hours of the day when our student chose to sleep. As his sleep clock appeared to be totally erratic, we expected his choice of sleep times to be random. Imagine our surprise when we found that amid the "chaos" there was a clear regularity to his daytime sleep routine. Significantly, he tended to go to sleep during two time windows—either from 4 to 6 P.M. or from 4 to 6 A.M. During the entire four-year examination period, he slept at the "normal" hour of 10 or 11 P.M. on only four occasions.

At this period, we were also studying the times when road accidents frequently occur owing to sleepy drivers. We chanced upon further evidence showing that the craving for sleep increased dramatically during these same windows. More than ten thousand serious road accidents occur in Israel annually. Although only 0.6–0.8 percent of them result from a driver falling asleep, casualties and property damage are three times more severe than those associated with accidents not caused by driver sleepiness.

To test whether there are "high-risk" hours for accidents caused by driver sleepiness, we checked the police computer. Analysis showed that most accidents occurred in two daily windows: 3–6 A.M. and 3–6 P.M.— close to the windows found in the student whose sleep clock had been disrupted. It is not surprising that the risk of falling asleep at the wheel and causing an accident increases strongly in the early hours of the morning. The personal experience of many people shows us that the need for sleep at that time increases, thus endangering the driver. Yet, the fact that the chances of falling asleep at the wheel in the afternoon were greater than those during the early evening hours only strengthened our feeling that something happens to the sleep-wakefulness mechanism dur-

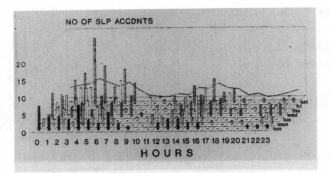

NO OF SLP ACCDNTS

HOURS

Fig. 19. Distribu-
tion of car acci-
dents in Israel
caused by falling
asleep at the wheel,
by hour of day and
day of week

ing those hours. This "something" intensifies the need for sleep. We
assumed that the activation of the sleep mechanisms during those hours
is not dependent on the level of fatigue or a lack of sleep, but probably
expresses an internal change in the working of the sleep clock. This
conclusion seems to be borne out by the custom, well established in many
countries, of taking an afternoon nap, or siesta.

## "SLEEP GATES" AND "FORBIDDEN ZONES FOR SLEEP"

How can we prove that the propensity for sleep varies regularly throughout the day? One way is to allow people to fall asleep many times during
the day and measure the time taken to fall asleep at those times.

The first scientist to use a test of the speed of falling asleep for
determining the propensity for sleep was Prof. Mary Carskadon of Brown
University, who, as a student of Dement, Kleitman's successor, is a third-
generation sleep researcher. Carskadon tested the daily sleepiness levels
of subjects who tried to fall asleep every two hours in a dark, soundproof
room between 10 A.M. and 8 P.M. This test has become known in the
literature as the multiple sleep latency test (MSLT). After a seven-hour
night's sleep, the average time taken to fall asleep was approximately
fifteen to seventeen minutes, and in many instances the subjects did not
manage to fall asleep at all. In contrast, sleep-deprived subjects fell
asleep very quickly, within five to seven minutes, as did people suffering
from an increased need to sleep or various other disorders.

According to Carskadon's reports, subjects tended to fall asleep more
quickly during the afternoon and had difficulty falling asleep during the

evening. Yet the measurement of sleep latency every two hours is not enough to ensure a precise description of the changes in sleep propensity throughout the day. We therefore developed a somewhat innovative research technique at the Technion, which has assisted us greatly in the discernment of daily changes in sleep propensity.

In a typical experiment, subjects arrived at the laboratory in the evening and spent the night awake. They were under the constant, strict supervision of the experimenters, who allowed them no possibility of falling asleep. At 7 o'clock the following morning, the subjects were shown into their bedrooms and asked to try to fall asleep within seven minutes. During this period brain waves, eye movements, and muscle tonus were duly recorded. When the seven minutes had elapsed, they were asked to leave their bedrooms for thirteen minutes, irrespective of whether they had fallen asleep or not. At 7:20 A.M. the experiment was repeated, and then every twenty minutes until 7 the following morning. The subjects were thus allowed seventy-two attempts at falling asleep over a period of twenty-four hours, so that the daily sleepiness pattern of each subject could be drawn according to his or her sleep latency in each of the seventy-two trials.

Although we did not advertise for volunteers, our "7/13" experiments were not short of candidates. Rumor of the impending experiment spread through the Technion like wildfire and the laboratory was flooded with students hopeful of being accepted for a study in which they were paid to sleep! Some dubbed themselves "sleep guinea pigs" and participated in the experiment four or five times during their studies. As subjects spent the night prior to the experiment without sleep, it might have been expected that they would have fallen asleep easily the next day, even though they would have been allowed to sleep for only a few minutes. The results of the 7/13 experiments, however, were more complex and displayed great variations in subjects' ability to fall asleep. We found that there were three windows during the day in which spontaneous changes in sleep latency occurred: in the afternoon, in the evening, and at night.

It was to be expected that the subjects would fall asleep quickly at night and in the early hours of the morning, and indeed at that time of day it was sometimes very difficult to get the subjects out of bed at the end of their allotted seven-minute sleep period. It was even harder to

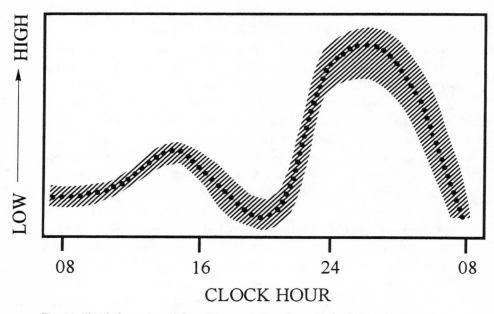

Fig. 20. The daily pattern of sleep "propensity" as shown in the 7/13 study

keep them awake for the thirteen minutes before the next attempt at falling asleep. Likewise, in the light of what we already knew about falling asleep in the afternoon and from our findings on road accidents related to driver drowsiness, we were not surprised to discover that sleepiness also showed an increase in the afternoons, even in subjects who did not usually sleep during those hours. The biggest surprise, however, was in the change in the level of sleepiness during the evening. Despite their tiredness and accumulated lack of sleep, our subjects found it difficult to fall asleep in the evening. Some could not fall asleep even once between 8 and 10 P.M., but the moment the door was closed behind them at 10 o'clock, they fell asleep, and from that time on they fell asleep quickly every time. It was as though a "sleep gate" which had been locked during the evening had suddenly opened wide. Indeed, this is the term we use to describe this sudden change from a high level of alertness to one of extreme sleepiness. The period preceding the gate, during which the subjects found it so difficult to fall asleep, is called the "forbidden zone for sleep." It correlated precisely not only with the hours in which the student with the sleep "clock" avoided going to sleep but also with the lowest point in sleep-related car accidents which occurred during the evening.

Is there any evidence that opening the sleep gate is correlated with a concomitant change in brain activity? Recent findings from Harvard may have proved just that. In the January 12, 1996 issue of *Science* magazine, a research group headed by Clifford Saper reported that they have found a master switching mechanism for sleep in the rat's hypothalamus. When the switch—a tiny cluster of nerve cells in the anterior hypothalamus—is turned on, all brain cells involved in arousal are shut down. Conversely, when the switch is turned off, the brain wakes up. This mechanism, however, is not responsible for making people drowsy and starts them on the somnolent slide. The newly discovered mechanism functions as an "all or nothing" phenomenon. It is tempting to suggest that opening of the sleep gate as revealed by the 7/13 paradigm results from a change in the activity of the hypothalamic switching-on mechanism. At that particular time, perhaps under the influence of the brain sleep clock, people's threshold of activation becomes much lower, thus enabling a fast and smooth transition from wake to sleep.

# From Sun Clocks
# to Biological Clocks

By this point, I hope the reader is convinced that sleep rhythm is a result of brain activity and not of extraneous factors. Let us now take a short detour to examine the new and thrilling research field of chronobiology, or the study of biological rhythms, which was developed during the second half of the twentieth century.

For someone born into a world in which day and night alternate every twenty-four hours, it is very difficult to imagine other forms of life. Indeed, if the earth did not rotate on its axis, then one side would always be light while the other remained in darkness. Vast differences would doubtless exist between those who lived in the light and those in the dark, and two animal kingdoms would be created: creatures of the light and creatures of the dark. Neither would be able to exist in the other's environment.

The earth's rotation sentences all the inhabitants of the planet to eternal alternating light and darkness. Three forms of adjustment to earth rotation developed during the evolutionary process: that of nocturnal animals whose activity begins with the setting of the sun; that of daylight animals who come to life at sunrise; and that of animals who are active twice a day, close to sunrise and sunset.

Existence is jeopardized by blind obedience to environmental conditions. In winter, for example, when the sunlight is unable to penetrate the clouds for days on end, and in the absence of any signal for the start of the day's activity, daylight animals are likely to starve to death. In order to break away from this total dependence upon environmental rotation, endogenous biological clocks were developed during the evolutionary process. These are neuro-mechanisms capable of measuring time and signaling the organism to commence or cease its activity periodically. Biological clocks allow the organism to do the right thing at the right time with great flexibility. They also perform other functions in which close coordination with the external environment is required. Biological clocks play an active part in the navigational mechanism of migrating birds, as well as in the way animals measure the length of the day in order to forecast the best time for mating.

In light of all this, it is quite amazing that recognition of the importance of biological clocks took such a long time. The ancient physicians were well aware of the existence of the cyclic changes in both the healthy and sick human body. They sought an explanation for this periodicity in the movements of heavenly bodies. Hippocrates, the father of Greek medicine, concluded that a physician should not be allowed to treat patients until he had proved his familiarity with the movements of the planets, for "the rising and setting of the stars has a great effect on sickness."

Although the first scientific experiment which showed that the origins of biological cycles were internal and not external was conducted in the eighteenth century, its importance did not gain recognition until more than two hundred years later. In 1728 Jean de Mairan, a French astronomer, reported to the Royal Academy of Science in Paris on an experiment he had conducted on the movement of the leaves of the mimosa, a plant that opens its leaves during the day and closes them at night. De Mairan moved his plant into a completely darkened room and found that it continued to open and close its leaves as though it were still exposed to alternate light and darkness, and he thus demonstrated the circadian cycle for the first time. In his report, de Mairan tried to link this phenomenon with the sleep of patients who were bedridden for long periods and who continued to sleep and awaken in a regular rhythm, but his hypothesis did not make a great impression. More than thirty years elapsed before someone else tried to repeat de Mairan's experiment, and irrefutable proof that the source of the leaf movement rhythm was in the plant itself came more than a century later. In this experiment, under conditions of complete darkness, the plant opened its leaves two or three hours earlier every day, showing a cycle which was shorter than twenty-four hours. It will be remembered that with humans in isolation, the sleep-wakefulness rhythm is extended to twenty-five hours and sometimes even longer. Although interest in the subject of biological rhythms did not wane completely, only a few people were aware of these experiments, the findings of which remained buried in dusty archives.

Until the twentieth century, physicians were pretty much the only people who showed any interest in the existence of biological rhythms. They tried to explain the strange tendency of all sorts of illnesses to appear in cycles, which were sometimes surprisingly precise. Yet most physicians were satisfied with a description of the symptoms, without trying to examine their source. The first researchers to investigate the source of biological rhythms were those who systematically measured various physiological functions which occurred over a period of twenty-four hours. For example, anyone who has ever studied the function of the kidney would have to take into account that the volume of urine changes constantly from morning to night, irrespective of the volume of liquid ingested at those times. One of the first books on the wonders of the biological clock was published in the nineteenth century by an English physician who developed instruments for the measurement of urine and its constituents, and also of the constituents of exhaled air. The same physician, Edward Smith, was among the first to conduct controlled experiments in order to understand the way biological clocks worked, for he accorded them considerable significance in the regulation of physiological processes.

As we saw in Chapter 5, Jürgen Aschoff, who has possibly contributed more than any other researcher to the study of the workings of the biological clock which controls sleep and wakefulness, admitted that he was drawn to the study of biological clocks almost involuntarily. He began to pay attention to them only after it became clear to him that wide variations in body temperature occur throughout the day, variations which cannot be explained by changes in environmental or experimental conditions.

The number of researchers working on biological clocks has increased constantly over the years, and today they are found all over the world. There are also three scientific journals devoted exclusively to biological rhythms.

Research has shown us that the body contains multiple systems which function cyclically. The durations of the cycles vary drastically: the heart, the cycle of which is measured in seconds; the REM sleep cycle, which lasts for some ninety minutes; the circadian-daily cycle; and monthly and yearly cycles which regulate reproductive behavior.

## BODY TEMPERATURE AND THE SLEEP CLOCK

Although many rhythms have a similar cycle duration, this does not necessarily indicate the presence of a single mechanism. Even when the two rhythms that share the same periodicity appear to be synchronized, it does not mean that they are controlled by a single "clock." In a natural environment, all the clock "hands" are influenced by the geophysical cycles. To study the true characteristics of the clocks, the organism should be isolated from the environmental time cues. The relationship between sleep-wakefulness and body temperature rhythms can serve as a notable example of this.

The first to measure body temperature for medical purposes was a sixteenth-century Venetian physician, Sanctorius Sanctorius, who invented the first known thermometer from a tube connected to a glass bulb containing a fluid. When the bulb was placed in his hand or put into the patient's mouth, the fluid in the tube rose, thus enabling the physician to observe any changes in body temperature. Although the physician was now able to estimate his patient's chances of recovery, the real significance of body temperature changes was locked in the prevailing concept of sickness at the time—an imbalance between the four corporeal fluids constituting the human body.

The breakaway from Greek medicine changed medical views regarding body temperature measurement. The concept of each illness having its individual body temperature gave way to an approach which held that body temperature was a general sign of sickness and disease. We have no authentic information as to who was the first to notice that the body temperature of healthy humans is not constant but fluctuates throughout the day. However, it is almost certain that the discovery was made around the time when thermometers were first used for medical purposes. The first books on medicine devoted to medical temperature measurement, published in the nineteenth century, contain clear references to the fact that body temperature reaches its peak during the afternoon or early evening and then drops to its lowest point toward awakening in the early hours of the morning. The difference between the high and low points can be as large as a whole degree (37.40° to 36.40°C, or 99.3° to 97.5°F), albeit in most cases the fluctuation is not more than half a degree. Changes in the daily rhythm of body temperature do not result from changes in the ambient temperature during transition from day to night or from muscular activity during the day. The rhythm continues even when a person remains in the same position, is sleep-deprived for an extended period, or fasts.

It is sometimes amazing to find how deeply rooted is the belief that a change of body temperature results solely from sickness. In the course of my lectures on body temperature rhythm to medical students, I have frequently encountered skepticism and even total disbelief. I even asked one class to measure their body temperature every two hours during an entire day, simply because several students were unconvinced by the findings I had presented.

What happens to body temperature rhythm in a time-free environment? To the great joy of the early researchers, the changes in body temperature rhythm followed the changes in the sleep-wakefulness rhythm very closely. The body temperature cycle periodicity was lengthened to exactly the same extent as the sleep-wakefulness rhythm, and this indicated the possibility that a single biological clock was responsible for both rhythms. In addition to the lengthening of the cycle, there was also a change in the coordination between the two. People in a natural environment go to sleep when their body temperature curve begins its daily descent, but it is still some hours away from its nadir, which appears in the early hours of the morning, around 4 or 5 A.M., just before the end of sleep. In isolation, on the other hand, a change occurs in the daily nadir: it moves to the beginning of sleep and a subject elects to go to sleep when his or her body temperature is at its lowest daily point. Some scientists viewed this as a logical explanation of the change which had occurred in the subject's sleep rhythm. Somehow, the subject sensed the drop in his body temperature and this was an internal signal for the choice of sleeping time.

Scientific theories, logical though they might be, are propounded only so that they may be disproved. As data on sleep-wakefulness and body temperature rhythms in isolation accumulated, it became clear that a single clock could not possibly control both. During periods of isolation lasting over two or three weeks, the two rhythms separated and each one maintained its own periodicity. It was impossible to forecast the time of separation; would it be a few days or even weeks after the beginning of the isolation? And yet a regularity in the results of the separation could have been found quite easily.

In every case of separation, the periodicity of the sleep-wakefulness rhythm was extended in comparison with the periodicity of the cycle prior to separation—from 26 to 27 hours, for example—while the periodicity of the body temperature cycle was shortened from 26 to 24.5 or 25 hours. These findings led Richard Kronauer, a Harvard mathematician, and the chronobiologist Charles Czeisler to assume that two different biological clocks controlled sleep-wakefulness and body temperature. In a natural environment, both had a periodicity of 24 hours and both were coordinated with natural conditions of light and darkness, but during the initial period of isolation they were coordinated so that their joint cycle was closer to body temperature cycle periodicity, and sleep always began when body temperature was at its lowest point. At a later stage of the isolation period they separate, and each adopts a periodicity of its own.

It was later found that each of the clocks is responsible for an additional number of systems. The body temperature clock supervises the secretion of the hormone cortisol, the secretion of potassium from the kidneys, and the appearance of REM sleep, while the sleep clock is responsible for the secretion of the growth hormone. As mentioned earlier, the growth hormone is secreted during the first part of the night and cortisol during the second part. As the duration of the joint cycle is closer to that of the body temperature cycle during the initial period of isolation, Kronauer and Czeisler termed the biological clock which controls body temperature "the strong oscillator," and that which controls sleep-wakefulness was dubbed "the weak oscillator."

## INTERNAL CLOCK ENTRAINMENT

The basic characteristics of the human sleep-wakefulness clock and that of activity-rest in animals (the cyclic periodicity of which also deviates from twenty-four hours) call for a daily adjustment of cycle periodicity in order to adapt it to the geophysical day. How is this adjustment made?

The most important environmental factor influencing the function of the biological clocks is the alternation of day and night, or of light and darkness. The importance of light is so great that in primitive animals the biological clock responsible for their activity-rest cycle is located in the eye itself. In birds, whose biological clock has shifted from the eye to the brain, the clock contains light-sensitive nerve cells, and it may be assumed that these are survivors from the time when the eye performed the function of the biological clock. Mammals possess a special nerve path along which information on the level of environmental light is transmitted from the retina to the biological clock, which is located in the area of the hypothalamus. This path is separate from that along which information is transmitted from the retina to the visual cerebral cortex.

Light, therefore, is of tremendous importance to the entrainment of internal clocks. In nocturnal animals, for example, the activity-rest rhythms can be entrained to suit the twenty-four-hour cycle by exposing them to short flashes of light at extremely low intensities. A radical example of this is bats, whose biological clock can be entrained to adjust to a cycle different from twenty-four hours by exposing them, at predetermined intervals, to a single flash of light lasting for less than one-thousandth of a second!

Unlike the findings of the influence of light on the biological clocks of animals, the first studies on humans revealed that their biological clock was not sensitive to light. Exposing humans in isolation to alternate light and darkness by switching table lamps on and off had no effect on the sleep-wakefulness clock. The researchers' conclusions were that, unlike in animals, the most significant factors in the entrainment of human internal clocks were social in nature. Only in recent years has it become clear that this conclusion was erroneous, for human biological clocks respond to light in exactly the same way as those of animals, the only difference being the required light intensity. It was found that a much higher light intensity was required in order to influence the rhythm of the human biological clock.

This discovery came about only after it became clear that a special hormone, melatonin, which is produced in the pineal gland deep in the brain, acts as an intermediary between light and the biological clocks.

## THE PINEAL GLAND AND THE DARKNESS HORMONE

The story of the study of the pineal gland and melatonin, the hormone it produces, is extraordinary. Until the mid-twentieth century, researchers concurred only on the fact that the human pineal gland tends to calcify early and can thus be used as a reference point in skull X rays. As the pineal is the only single gland located between the two hemispheres of the brain, French philosopher René Descartes thought that it was the site of the "rational mind." Conventional wisdom held that the pineal gland was an evolutionary throwback from an earlier developmental stage, but this did not satisfy Mark Altschule, a Harvard doctor, and he decided systematically to study all the scientific literature on the gland. After reviewing more than eighteen hundred articles in twelve languages, he realized that there was evidence that the pineal gland was linked to at least three processes: genital function, of the ovaries in females and of the testes in males; the lightening of skin pigmentation in animals; and a possible control of brain activity. Altschule and his colleague, Julian Kitay, published their findings in a book which signaled a turning point in the status of the pineal gland.

At the same time as Altschule's efforts—but totally unrelated to them—Aaron Lerner, a Yale dermatologist who was interested in factors which affected skin pigmentation, came across a scientific report on the effects of pineal gland extract on skin pigmentation in frogs and decided to try to isolate its active compound. In 1956, after extracting material from some 250,000 glands, he succeeded in isolating the active compound, which he named melatonin, as it is derived from the neurotransmitter serotonin and affects melanin in the skin.

Mark Altschule's book and Lerner's discovery of melatonin became the basis of modern pineal gland research, and later one discovery came fast on the heels of another. After a number of years, the pineal gland and melatonin became a focal point of interest for researchers in many and varied fields.

It appeared that the pineal gland was the transducer which translated environmental changes in light and darkness to physiological and hormonal changes in the body through the production of melatonin. As the hormone is produced in darkness and its production ceases during the daylight hours, melatonin levels in the bloodstream reflect the number of daylight and nighttime hours. During the long winter nights, the level of melatonin in the blood is high, while it is low during the short summer nights. Thus we are better able to understand the relationship between the pineal gland and the sex organs, as a high melatonin level retards genital development. Therefore, during the winter months when the days are short and many wild animals spend much of their time in darkness, the melatonin level in the bloodstream is very high and genital development is repressed. Once the days begin to lengthen in the spring and summer, and environmental conditions are conducive to breeding, the melatonin level is gradually reduced, the sex organs are able to function, and mating and breeding takes place. The old saying "In the spring a young man's fancy lightly turns to thoughts of love" has a solid physiological and hormonal foundation. It is therefore not surprising that animals living in the polar regions, which are notable for radical changes in the duration of the day in both summer and winter, have an especially large pineal gland.

Laboratory experiments have shown that animals can be deceived by changes in their cage lighting. If they are exposed to long or short days, they will behave as though it were "winter" or "summer" according to their exposure to light. Chicken farmers who light their coops during the night in order to increase egg production have been using this subterfuge to fool their birds for years. The effect of melatonin on skin pigmentation is also linked to the entire gamut of physiological changes which accompany the sexual behavior of animals. During the mating season, many animals change the color of their skin or fur in order to increase their sexual attraction.

In view of the evolutionary importance of light, it seemed that human beings were unusual by virtue of their lack of sensitivity to it. Some tried to ascribe this phenomenon to human sexual behavior, which is not affected by the seasons of the year or the length of the day. The breakthrough came with the discovery that melatonin production in human beings is suppressed if they are exposed to particularly bright light.

Al Lewy, a psychiatrist at the National Institutes of Health in the United States, now in Portland, Oregon, has studied the effects on melatonin levels in humans of exposure to light at varying intensities during the night. His findings showed that exposure to light suppresses the production of melatonin in humans, and indeed, the required light intensity was much higher than that needed for the suppression of melatonin production in other animals.

Illumination intensity is measured in a unit called a lux. We are exposed to greatly varying light intensities during the course of a normal day. The intensity of daylight, for example, is some hundred thousand lux, while that of the reading lamp on our bedside table does not exceed one hundred lux. Our visual system has special sensors for vision at both high and low light intensities, and it works well under both sets of conditions. But the pineal gland cannot "see" low-intensity light at all, and the minimum light intensity required to suppress the production of melatonin is twenty-five hundred lux. Light of this intensity is measured several minutes after sunrise on a clear day, at a distance of one meter from our bedroom window.

Lewy's findings showed that exposure to twenty-five hundred lux or more not only suppresses melatonin production but also changes the human biological clock. Exposure to bright light during the evening delays the daily body temperature nadir which occurs during the early hours of the morning, and delays sleep time. We shall see that exposure to bright light can be used to reset maladjusted biological clocks which are the cause of sleep and wakefulness disorders.

Is the secretion of melatonin therefore linked to the control of the human sleep-wakefulness rhythm? There is some proof of this. In a study we conducted at a blind children's school in Jerusalem, we examined the connection between the daily secretion of melatonin and sleep disorders in young blind people. We found that boys and girls who suffered from sleep disorders also showed an abnormal melatonin secretion pattern; the peak of melatonin secretion did not occur during the night, as it does with sighted people, but during the day. The sleep rhythm of one of the boys who suffered from severe sleep disorders and who was treated with melatonin improved beyond recognition.

Later, Orna Tzischinsky, a doctoral student in my laboratory, obtained evidence that the opening of the sleep gate at night in normal-sighted young adults may be mediated by the nocturnal rise in melatonin secretion, since she found a close relationship between the two events. Furthermore, exogenously administered melatonin during the early evening could advance the opening of the gate to earlier times. These experimental findings suggest that secretion of melatonin may play a much bigger role in the regulation of sleep than was considered previously.

We may sum up by saying that human internal clocks are affected by and coordinated with social factors and the environmental alternation of light and darkness. Every day, the internal clock resets itself in accordance with the external environment. By exposing the internal clocks to bright light, their behavior can be changed; exposure to light during the evening delays both sleeping time and the low point in the daily rhythm of body temperature. Exposure to bright light during the morning hours has the opposite effect, advancing sleeping time and the low point in the daily rhythm of body temperature. In such a way the light-dark cycle maintains its control over the endogenous biological clock.

# Dreams

## *Creatures of the Brain*

Since the dawn of history, humankind has been preoccupied with the source and significance of dreams. Primitive societies perceived their dreams as an integral part of their lives. A North American Indian who dreamed that he had been bitten by a snake would treat himself for snakebite immediately upon waking. Some tribes believed that the source of dreams was in the soul, which left the body to roam the world during sleep and which signaled its return when the sleeper awoke. It was therefore forbidden to wake a sleeper suddenly, for the soul might not have managed to return to his body. In ancient religions, from the Sumerians and Babylonians to the Greeks, dreams were perceived as a means of communication between the gods and mortals. Dreams were the instrument for prophesying and understanding the intentions and desires of the gods. A despairing Saul complained to the prophet Samuel, "and God is departed from me, and answereth me no more, neither by prophets nor by dreams" (1 Samuel 28:15).

People made pilgrimages from all over the Middle East to special ritual sites, the most famous of which were the temples at Delphi in Greece and Memphis in Egypt, in order to dream. The pilgrims slept in the temple precincts in the hope that the gods, or the souls of the departed, would appear in their dreams. In the morning, the high priestess would interpret the dreams and instruct the dreamers as to what action they should take. In later times, people believed that dreams resulted from the effects of physical or external stimuli on the sleeping brain and therefore perceived dreams as having a diagnostic value insofar as the physical condition of the dreamer was concerned. Interest in dreams increased, especially in the nineteenth century, when the dream began to be viewed as a connecting link between normal thought and the hallucinations of the deranged and insane. There can be no doubt that interest in dreams reached its peak after Freud accorded dreams cardinal importance in psychoanalytic theory. In his book *The Interpretation of Dreams,* published in 1900, Freud claimed that dreams are "the royal road to a knowledge of the unconscious activities of the mind."

Freud and psychoanalysis are also largely responsible for the popular image and significance of the dream in the twentieth century. The patient lying on the psychiatrist's couch while relating his dreams has become the subject of innumerable jokes and cartoons, but according to Freud it is not enough to simply relate the dream, for the patient's account is, in fact, a cover or camouflage of the dream's latent content, and that can be exposed only by psychoanalysis.

## REM SLEEP: A WINDOW ON THE WORLD OF DREAMS

The discovery of REM sleep by Aserinsky and Kleitman in 1953, coupled with the fact that waking from this sleep stage is bound up with a clear and detailed report of a dream, allowed researchers, for the first time, to identify the moment of the "dream." It is not difficult to imagine the excitement that gripped those interested in dreams once it became clear that dreams did not occur at random throughout the night, but at a specific and easily identifiable stage of sleep. The discovery of REM sleep brought psychiatrists and psychologists much closer to the sources of the dream itself, so it was hardly surprising that the majority of sleep researchers who rushed to their laboratories in order to study what transpired during REM sleep were those whose main interest lay in dreams. They no longer had to rely on their patients' memories in order to learn about their dreams; by waking them up at the correct time they were able to hear the dreams firsthand.

The technique was extremely simple: all the researcher had to do was to remain alert throughout the night and observe the instruments recording the subject's brain waves, eye movements, and muscle tonus. At the precise moment that the recording sheet showed the characteristic configuration of REM sleep, the researcher had to rouse the patient. As we have already seen, this configuration is easily identifiable and almost unmistakable. Several minutes after the appearance of REM sleep, the researcher would open the bedroom door, quietly call the subject's name and, when he or she awoke, ask, "Did you dream about anything?" It was only some years later, for reasons that will soon become apparent, that the question was revised to, "Did anything cross your mind?" And indeed, this wait for the onset of REM sleep was usually not in vain. In 80–85 percent of the cases, the subjects awakening from REM sleep were able to provide a clear and detailed report of their dream.

So if dreams occur during REM sleep, why are we unable to remember them every time we awaken from it? After the subject awakens from REM sleep, although the story of a dream is stored in a readily accessible memory bank, it remains there for a very short time. If we divert the subject's attention from the story of a dream or delay its telling, then the "memory banks" close and traces of the dream will become blurred. In many cases, therefore, people awaken from sleep with a clear feeling that they have had a dream but are unable to remember anything about it. This also explains why it is easier to remember dreams after being awakened suddenly. When people wake up gradually over a few minutes, their attention may drift and the dream story rapidly fades.

The majority of studies conducted in sleep laboratories during the 1960s dealt with planned awakenings from REM sleep in order to obtain dream reports. However, as more and more dreams were collated in the laboratory, it became clear that laboratory dreams were vastly different from those reported during treatment on the psychiatrist's couch. Laboratory dreams were much shorter, less "strange," and poorer in content than those reported in psychology and psychiatry literature. Most of them dealt with everyday matters, and a few included strange details which deviated from normal thinking while awake. The picture which was formed of the content of dreams showed that the majority were based upon the same images and events to which we are exposed in our everyday lives. People dream about subjects that are close to their hearts: lawyers dream about courtrooms, judges, and criminals; doctors dream about operating rooms, hospital corridors, and white-clad nurses; students dream about lecturers and examinations. It is therefore not surprising to find that those who dream about matters of paramount national and global concern are usually politicians! Fred Snyder, a veteran American sleep researcher, summed up his rich experience in the study of the contents of dreams thus: "Our findings on the contents of dreams show that they are a true reflection of our waking lives."

Some explained this phenomenon by the interrogation method used. The need to awaken the sleeper in the middle of REM sleep in order not to miss the dream is reminiscent of watching a movie to the middle without seeing the end. Others explained it thus: the spontaneously remembered dream is usually the last one of the night and is probably exceptional in comparison with those dreamed early in the night.

Is there, then, a difference between the dream reports received from the early REM period of the night and those of the later periods? It was indeed found that there is a development in dream character during the night, from one dream period to the next. Usually, after awakening from the first dream period, the report is brief, deals with the present, and in most cases lacks a plot or central characters. The reports become richer in detail and plot as awakening is effected from REM sleep late at night. Dream reports made in the early hours of the morning are richer in detail, central characters, and feelings, and, compared with dreams from the first half of the night, they tend to deal more with the dreamer's early childhood. These dreams from the last hours of the night, prior to awakening, are those which are remembered spontaneously.

## DREAMS, THOUGHTS, OR HALLUCINATIONS?

When Aserinsky and Kleitman first discerned rapid eye movements in sleep, it was only natural that they should assume that the movements were connected to dreaming. Dement examined this assumption in the simplest and most direct way: he wakened the subjects when they moved their eyes and asked them whether they had been dreaming. In 1957, Dement and Kleitman published the first article describing the connection between rapid eye movements and dreams. Their subjects reported on clear, detailed dreams after 152 out of 191 awakenings from REM sleep. However, after a total of 160 wakenings from other sleep stages, only eleven times did they manage to report a dream. This 80 percent success rate in recalling REM sleep dreams was substantiated by other studies. They led to the conclusion that dreams occur solely during REM sleep and that the partial remembering of them that occurred during other sleep stages were fragments of dreams from the previous REM sleep, which later materialized in adjacent sleep stages.

Not everyone agreed that dreams occur exclusively during REM sleep. Some claimed that this apparent relationship was a result of a methodological error. When awakening from other sleep stages, subjects were unconsciously guided by the researchers to give a negative reply to the question "Did you dream?" When people wake up and are asked this question, their replies will depend, among other things, on their conceptions of the term *dream*. Although it is widely accepted that a dream is a kind of cognitive activity which takes place during sleep, the definition of this activity may vary radically from person to person. There are those for whom a dream is every cognitive activity which occurs during sleep, irrespective of its content. Others report on a dream only when the cognitive activity includes events deviating from day-to-day reality. It is probable that people who awaken from sleep stages other than REM sleep deny having "dreamed" because the experience they underwent did not fit their conception of a dream.

David Foulkes, who worked first at the University of Chicago and then at the University of Wyoming, was the first to test this possibility scientifically. He reworded the question put to the subjects; instead of asking them, "Did you dream?" he asked "Did anything cross your mind before awakening?" Thus, the subject's reply was not limited to dreams. Indeed, Foulkes's studies and those of later researchers showed a far higher percentage of reports after awakening from sleep stages other than REM sleep, compared with the first laboratory studies, which had been confined to reports of actual visual dreams. When a comparison was made between reports of REM sleep and those of other sleep stages, it became clear that there was a vast difference in their character. Subjects who awakened from sleep other than REM sleep reported in most cases on their thoughts, fragments of thoughts, or fragments of ideas. These reports differed greatly from REM sleep reports, which were usually exemplified by the development of a plot and a plethora of details and feelings. For example, a student who spent a number of nights in the Technion Sleep Laboratory made the following report after awakening from sleep stage 2 at the beginning of the night: "The thought of the math exam we had yesterday crossed my mind." A completely identical subject appeared in the report made by another student who awoke from his third REM sleep: "I dreamed that I was sitting in the Ullman Building studying math. I knew the lecturer but I was unable to identify any of the other people around me. My pocket calculator was on the desk and for some reason I tried to spread mayonnaise and ketchup on it just as you woke me."

The preponderance of reports after waking up from stages of sleep other than REM was explained by some researchers as evidence that the stream of consciousness never ceases. The brain produces cognitive activity in all stages during sleep and wakefulness. The reason that reports after awakenings from REM sleep are richer in detail and plot than reports after waking up from stage 2, they claimed, is that retrieving the cognitive activities is dependent on cortical arousal. Higher levels of arousal, such as in REM sleep, are associated with more details being reported.

Another form of cognitive activity connected with transitional sleep, or sleep stage 1, is called "hypnagogic hallucinations." During the falling-asleep process, which is gradual and continues for several minutes, a great change occurs in the thought process. From the focused thought of wakefulness, thought becomes more and more associative and less focused until it becomes pictorial. The pictures may change rapidly, jumping from subject to subject and from one view to another. In many cases there is a clear continuity between the last sensory impressions experienced immediately before falling asleep and the contents of the hypnagogic hallucinations. As we shall see, these hallucinations can be altered by the use of external stimuli.

## THE SOURCES OF DREAMS

What are the sources of dreams? Have the planned awakenings from REM sleep advanced our knowledge concerning the stuff dreams are made on? Freud claimed that the dream is nourished by the day's residues, those same unimportant pieces of information that were absorbed almost inadvertently during the day. So will the events of the past day appear in the following night's dreams? Not always.

The first researcher to note this phenomenon was the eminent French neurophysiologist Michel Jouvet. Having fought with the French Resis-

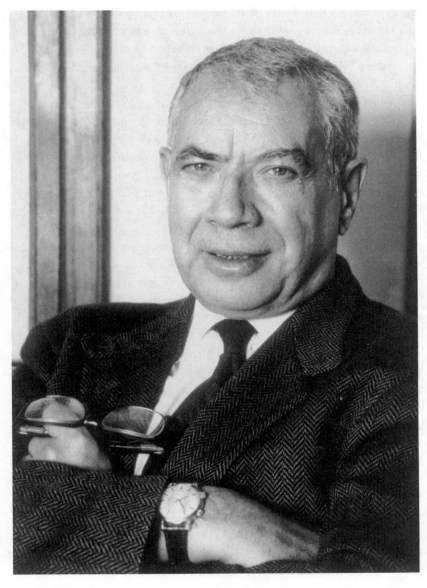

Fig. 21. Michel Jouvet

tance in the Second World War, Jouvet studied medicine at Lyons. He specialized in surgery, worked for some time as a neurosurgeon, and later performed amazingly precise surgery on laboratory animals in order to study sleep mechanisms. In 1991 the Technion awarded him an honorary doctorate in recognition of his achievements in the study of the neuro-physiological mechanisms which control sleep. For years Jouvet has faithfully recorded his own dreams every morning. So far he has collected more than twenty-five hundred. Many will wonder how it is possible to record so many dreams without resorting to the services provided by the sleep laboratory, but there is proof that the ability to remember can be enhanced by autosuggestion and a great deal of will power. Those who want to badly enough and who "decide" to remember their dreams can do so with a high degree of success.

When Jouvet began to analyze his dreams, he noted that the events which appeared in the story of his dreams were usually connected with the previous day or with something that had occurred during the previous week. This regularity became especially notable when Jouvet traveled abroad. As a lecturer who is in great demand, he flies all over the world from one scientific congress to another, and when he analyzed the dreams he had had during his travels, he realized that the new experiences he had undergone in new places usually did not appear immediately in the contents of the dream, but only a week after arrival at his destination. If, for example, he had flown to the United States, he continued to dream about subjects connected with Lyons and France for the first week, and only then would he begin to dream about events related to his new environment.

Jouvet's observations were later substantiated in two further studies using a large group of subjects. Both studies found that dreams were not only nourished by the previous day's events but also by events which had taken place six to eight days earlier. The Gulf War and the Scud missile attacks on Israel presented me with a unique opportunity of studying, indirectly, Jouvet's observations of the delay which occurs in the inclusion of the day's events in dream stories.

During the war, I was teaching a course to seventy students at the Technion's Faculty of Medicine. Immediately after the first missiles had hit Tel Aviv and Haifa, I asked the students to fill out a questionnaire about the quality of their sleep and to report on their dreams during the first week of the war. Despite the fact that only two or three days had passed since the first missile had hit Israel, only a few of the dreams reported dealt with the war. The questionnaire was again given to the students in the fifth week of the war, and then almost half of the dreams reported dealt directly or indirectly with the war. It is interesting to note that here, too, the contents of the dreams focused on the most worrying subjects of those days. As a result of Iraqi president Saddam Hussein's threats, the gas mask became an inseparable part of Israelis' standard equipment, and one of their greatest fears during the war was being caught in a missile attack without their masks. Indeed, the gas mask became the most common subject of dreams during the Gulf War. For example: "I dreamed that I was taking a shower when I heard the air-raid warning. I ran out of the shower dripping wet, but I could not decide whether I should first dry myself or put on my gas mask." I experienced a similar dream during the war. I was on a bus with my gas mask on the floor beside me. When I got off, I realized that I had left my mask behind on the bus, and just as I started to run after it, the air-raid warning siren suddenly sounded.

There is no convincing explanation of why the inclusion of the day's experiences in dream stories is delayed. Neither do we know whether the process is selective—in other words, whether the "dream machine" scans the memory banks and selects those items of information from which the dream is built, or whether the reason for the delay is the existence of a special memory bank, which is updated only once every few days and from which the dream details are selected. Is it possible, for example that, as in the theater, where there are permanent stage props that remain in place throughout the performance although the scenes and actors change, so some of our dreams rely on the same background memories. Much more research will be required to clarify these issues.

## THE DREAM OF THE SHEEP

All of the above notwithstanding, there are of course exceptions. In these cases, experiences and information from the last moments before sleep will appear in that night's dreams. It should be mentioned that, in many cases, these experiences are from the first night's sleep in the sleep laboratory. Sleep in the laboratory is no ordinary experience to be compared with sleeping away from home, at a hotel, or a summer camp. Subjects go to sleep connected to the recording instruments by means of electrodes attached to their head and face, with the clear knowledge that in the next room a group of impatient researchers is awaiting the first signs of REM sleep in order to awake them. These conditions are usually accompanied by a certain degree of fear and anxiety, especially on the first night in the lab. And indeed, when the subject is awakened from REM sleep on the first night, we usually find that a small part of the "sleep laboratory experience" has found its way into the dream story. The subject might dream about electrodes or the recording instruments, or even talk to the researcher in the dream. Laboratory-linked subjects or other tests which have become associatively linked to the sleep tests may also appear. As the following story will illustrate, dream stories frequently surprise the researchers themselves.

Some years ago, we prepared a television program on dreams and REM sleep, which was designed to describe the course of sleep as it is reflected on the recording instruments in the laboratory, and also to document the waking of a subject from REM sleep in order to hear a live report on a dream on camera. In order to film the program, the television team with all their equipment readied themselves for a night's stay in the Sleep Laboratory. Z.N., one of our senior "sleep technicians," volunteered for the role of guinea pig, and the camera followed his preparations for the sleep test. The interviewer opened the program with a few questions, such as, "Will you be able to fall asleep in the laboratory?" "What will you dream about?" "Are you worried about the test?" To the interviewer's great joy, Z.N. answered all the questions wittily and assured him that if he were unable to fall asleep, he would "count sheep until the morning."

Once the preparations had been completed, the camera followed Z.N. to the bedroom. On the wall of the corridor leading to the bedroom there hung a large painting by the noted Israeli artist Menashe Kadishman, called *Pink Sheep*. As Z.N. passed it, he jokingly remarked that the sheep he would count before going to sleep would probably be pink too. Happily for the television crew, who had no idea that sleep research usually required many hours of waiting, Z.N. did not need to count sheep and fell asleep immediately. The first REM sleep appeared as expected after about ninety minutes and, with the television camera following close behind, we approached Z.N.'s bed in order to record his dream report for posterity. He awoke easily, looked around in surprise at the strange faces and television cameras that surrounded him, and told us that we had interrupted him in the middle of a dream in which he was examining a patient lying in the hospital's emergency room. At this point in the story he hesitated for a moment, scratched his head and added, "The patient was no ordinary patient. It was a white sheep wearing a black bow tie. . . . I don't remember any more." It was only when I left the bedroom and went into the corridor that I saw Kadishman's pink sheep looking down at me from their place on the wall, and recognized the source of the dream. At that time, Z.N. was about to complete his medical studies, and in his dream he had put the sheep we had talked about in the few moments before he went to sleep into the emergency room, where, as part of his studies, he had spent many hours during the past month. I ascribed the addition of the black bow tie that the sheep wore around its neck to Z.N.'s highly developed sense of humor. It goes without saying that I found it extremely difficult to convince the viewers that Z.N.'s dream was completely authentic, and not an elaborate "setup."

Why do events which occur in the laboratory find their way into the dream story so quickly? And why do other events wait in line for a week? A possible answer may be found in the differences between spontaneously remembered dreams and those recalled after a planned awakening from REM sleep in the laboratory. Spontaneously remembered dreams are generally those from the last REM sleep of the night, and, as I have explained, the last dreams of the night deal with the dreamer's distant past, so there is little chance that they will include everyday experiences. On the other hand, with planned awakenings in the laboratory, dreams from the first REM sleep of the night can be remembered, dreams which deal with the dreamer's current experiences. According to this explanation, there is a prior delay in which everyday events merge with events from the dreamer's past. In contrast, the first dreams, which cannot be remembered in the morning, reflect what has occurred during the day.

# Alfred Maury and the Dream of the Guillotine

The use of electrophysiological recordings to identify the precise moment of the dream opened up a new method of study which assisted researchers in understanding the process through which dreams are formed. As I mentioned above, early scientists believed that dreams resulted from sensory impressions reaching the sleeping brain from the other parts of the body, or from the environment. In most cases, this claim was based on personal recounting. Sometimes noise, or another kind of environmental stimulus, penetrates REM sleep through the brain's blocking mechanisms and becomes intertwined in the dream story, usually associatively or "in disguise." For example, someone who remembers dreaming about "an ambulance that drove fast, sounding its siren loudly" may discover that he or she has been woken up by the strident ringing of the telephone. It is therefore probable that experiments on influencing the dream by the use of controlled stimuli during REM sleep can teach us something of the processes related to the formation of the dream.

One of the most fervent proponents of the relationship between physical stimuli and dreams was Alfred Maury, a nineteenth-century French scholar. Maury started to study medicine, and although he did not complete his studies, he was involved in French medical circles and contributed regularly to medical and scientific journals. His chief interest was dreams and their meaning. Maury was convinced that dreams were simply the result of physiological changes in the brain and nervous system, after they had received impressions from the sensory organs during sleep. His belief in physical influence on the brain during sleep was unassailable. "People forget that the mind is unable to grasp and sense without the body, just as the body is unable to digest food without the stomach," he argued.

Like many scientists of that era, Maury conducted experiments on himself. In his own words, he was the ideal dream researcher: "Very few people dream as rapidly and as much as I do. The traces of the majority of my dreams remain clear for many months . . . just as they were at the time I dreamt them." In the middle of the nineteenth century, these qualities, coupled with his love of the scientific approach, led Maury to conduct a series of experiments which were usually done in the following manner: He would lie on his bed or make himself comfortable in his armchair and try to fall asleep. His assistant would awaken him immediately after he had fallen asleep and Maury would make an on-the-spot report of what had crossed his mind after falling asleep. In some of the experiments, the assistant would use an assortment of stimuli—vocal sounds, tickling with a feather, or holding a candle close to Maury's feet—in order to test how they influenced the content of the dream.

A few of these stimuli were transformed into amusing fantasies in Maury's brain. When his assistant singed the soles of his feet with a candle, he reported that he had been captured by robbers who tried to discover where he had hidden his money by torturing him. Perfume which was dripped near his nose rapidly conveyed him to a Cairo spice merchant's shop, with all its colors and scents. He sometimes experienced exotic adventures which he was unable to reconstruct, or which, perhaps, he had no desire to relate!

Today we know that Maury studied not the dreams of REM sleep but hypnagogic hallucinations which bear a certain similarity to dreams. His reports, therefore, teach us that sensory impressions may indeed bear a real influence on hypnagogic hallucinations. As we shall soon see, this influence is far greater than the influence that sensory impressions have on the dream process itself. In his book *Le sommeil et les rêves* (Sleep and dreams), published in 1861, Maury summed up his observations: Dreams were nothing but an accompanying phenomenon of sensory impressions which were absorbed before and during sleep. He totally rejected the possibility that dreams had any meaning at all. In his view, the psychological significance of the dream was nothing but a reconstruction of impressions which reached the mind from the internal or external environment during sleep. These impressions became associated with childhood or other memories and thus created the story of the dream.

It is entirely possible that Maury's name would never have gained the prominence it did had it not been for one particular dream which left its mark for decades on beliefs regarding dreams and the manner in which they are created: the dream of the guillotine.

We do not know exactly when this dream occurred, but Maury said that it was when he lay ill one night and was cared for by his mother. In his dream, Maury saw himself at the time of the Reign of Terror during the French Revolution, "the symbol of which was the guillotine." After witnessing a large number of executions, he was summoned before the tribunal headed by Robespierre and Marat, which found him guilty of treason. He was then led to to the platform to join those about to be executed. His head was placed on the "lunette" and he saw the blade descend and hit his neck. He awoke in a great fright to discover that the canopy over his bed had fallen and the rod had landed upon his neck in the exact place the guillotine's blade would have hit had he indeed been beheaded. True to his belief that the source of the dream was in sensory impressions, he claimed that the entire dream of the guillotine had taken place in the extremely short time which had elapsed between the blow to his neck and his frightened awakening.

There can be no doubt that Maury's dream was influenced by the falling canopy, but we can say with the same degree of certainty that the dream was not caused by it. It is very probable that the conclusion of the dream would have been completely different had the canopy rod not fallen as it did. The dream itself, of the heroes of the French Revolution and the mass trials which inevitably ended with beheading, were most probably influenced by his childhood experiences and his admiration of the revolution's heroes. *Sleep and Dreams* contains descriptions of other dreams about the French Revolution, albeit far less dramatic than that of the guillotine. Even Sigmund Freud mentions the dream of the guillotine in *The Interpretation of Dreams*. True to his interpretations of the sources of the dream, Freud claims that the dream of the guillotine expressed Maury's hidden desire to die a hero's death as compensation for the frustration he had experienced as a failed politician.

## THE INDIFFERENCE OF THE DREAM MECHANISM

Thanks to the window opened on the world of dreams by the discovery of physiological REM sleep, it became possible to try to reconstruct Maury's experiments using a controlled procedure and to expose the sleeping subject to stimuli at the precise time of experiencing the dream. Many researchers tried to intervene during the course of the dream; some dripped cold water on the feet of the dreamers, while others made noises and sounded musical notes, or called the sleeper's name. Some made their subjects sleep with their eyelids taped open and then flashed brief bursts of light into their eyes during REM sleep. It was found that the contribution of external stimuli to the dream story was at best partial and even marginal. There was not a single case in which external stimulus became the central subject of the dream, and in many cases the stimulus did not appear in the dream at all. The disappointment stemming from the inability to divert the dreamer's attention from the creation of the dream to sensory information channels led Allan Rechtschaffen, one of the most eminent contemporary sleep researchers, to label the dream creation process "a single-minded process."

The possibility that stimuli originating in the body itself might have significant influence on the "editing" of dreams was also rejected. Micha Gross, who came from the University of Zurich to complete his doctoral studies in my laboratory, examined this question under controlled conditions. He studied the dreams of people who suffered from sleep apnea. This particular sleep disorder, which I shall discuss in detail in Chapter 19, is characterized by hundreds of suspensions of breathing, each lasting between twenty and forty seconds. There can be no doubt that suspension of breathing is indeed a powerful physical stimulus, the impressions of which quickly reach the brain. During the apnea, the blood oxygenation level drops and dramatic changes occur in both heart rate and blood pressure. These changes, which reach the brain, cause the sleeper to awaken and thus avoid suffocation. As sleep apnea appears during every stage of sleep, including REM sleep, we studied the dreams of sufferers from this syndrome and assumed that the dream stories of people who stop breathing while asleep would include details about suffocation, breathing difficulties, or fear and anxiety resulting from the stress to which they were subjected. It is difficult to describe our surprise when we found that not a single dream from among the hundreds dreamed by sleep apnea sufferers contained details, even indirectly, of breathing or suffocation. Neither were any significant dreams of explicit anxiety recorded. This firmly supported Rechtschaffen's claim regarding the single-mindedness of the dream creation mechanism during sleep. The mechanism is almost completely isolated from those areas of the brain whose function is sensory reception.

## REMEMBERING DREAMS—AND FORGETTING THEM

There is a consensus which holds that the chance of a person awakening from REM sleep and remembering his or her dream is approximately 80 percent. Nonetheless, not everyone has the same ability to remember dreams. There are those who are very good at it and remember their dreams every morning, while others are convinced that they did not dream at all because they are simply unable to remember even a single dream for months on end.

What causes these variations in the ability of people to remember dreams? As we have seen, remembering a dream is first and foremost conditional on the time of awakening from sleep. People who tend to wake up during REM sleep are more likely to remember their dreams than those who awaken from the other sleep stages. But the remembering of dreams also depends upon the depth of sleep. Those who sleep very deeply are less likely to remember their dreams than light sleepers, and in this context it is worthy of note that in our study of the dreams of sleep apnea sufferers, we found that they better remembered their dreams when they underwent repeated apneas than when they slept undisturbed as a result of successful treatment of their ailment. Their breathing disorder caused shallow sleep, and they were able to awaken from it more easily than after treatment, when their sleep became deeper and consequently their ability to remember their dreams diminished.

Memory is affected not only by the time we wake up in the morning and the depth of our sleep but also by our desire and readiness to remember dreams. People who underwent psychological treatment in the course of which they discussed their dreams suddenly discovered that

they began to remember their dreams increasingly. Subjects who participated in studies in which dreams were collected reported that their very
participation in the study increased their ability to remember. Therefore,
the best advice I can give people who want to remember dreams is to get
into bed after having made a firm decision to do so! They should keep a
notebook and pencil on their bedside table in order to record the story
of their dream immediately upon awakening, before the memory dissi-
pates.

The ability to recall a dream is also related to its content. We tend
to better remember dreams that are rich in content, unusual, strange, and
which arouse both our interest and emotions. Those that are brief, trivial,
and devoid of emotion tend to be swiftly forgotten. Just as we are able to
encourage the remembering of dreams, we can also encourage the forgetting of them. By the use of autosuggestion, people who suffer from
unpleasant dreams or nightmares can diminish the remembering of their
dreams. In the cases of people who have undergone traumatic experiences, the "erasing" of dreams can be so efficient that even awakening
the sleeper from REM sleep does not improve recollection.

## TRAUMA AND DREAMS

The term *post-traumatic dream* describes a particular type of dream
which is usually frightening and in which the dreamer compulsively returns to the place in which the trauma was experienced. Such dreams
are prevalent in those who have suffered war-related post-traumatic syndrome—for example, former prisoners of war or Holocaust survivors. A
post-traumatic dream reported in my laboratory which is etched upon my
memory is that of a fifty-five-year-old Holocaust survivor from Holland.
He spent several nights at the Technion Sleep Laboratory so that we could
discover the cause of his sleep disorders. When the technician aroused
him from REM sleep in order to record his dream, the subject related a
clear and detailed dream in a choked voice that was on the verge of tears.
His dream reconstructed a real-life incident which had occurred when
he was six years old. To save him from the Nazis, his parents had given
him up for adoption by a family of Christian neighbors who had made a
hurried departure from their own village to another distant one, where

the child's religion was unknown. Some weeks later, the boy was making his way along the village street when he bumped into one of his family's neighbors from his home village who knew that he was a Jew. As soon as he realized whom he had met, he froze in panic momentarily, and promptly fled to the nearby forest where he hid for several days. He was convinced that the neighbor would reveal his whereabouts to the Nazis. This meeting with the neighbor and their exchange of looks had appeared in his dreams almost every night for the next forty years. The dream was always terminated at the moment the neighbor was about to seize him in order to turn him over to the Gestapo. In his recounting of his dream, the fear and terror in his voice are difficult to describe. When he had finished his story, he thanked the technician for waking him up when he did, because he had "nearly been caught that time." Similar nightmares were recounted by many Holocaust survivors immediately after the war, but in some cases their frequency diminished as the years went by.

Over a period of many years, numerous Holocaust survivors complaining of sleep disorders were examined in the Technion Sleep Laboratory, yet only recently have we undertaken a systematic study of their dreams. It is no easy thing to explore the experiences and memories of those who lived through the hell of nazism, for there are many Holocaust survivors who avoid allowing others, even close relations, to share in those experiences. Hannah Kaminer, a clinical psychologist who questioned them as part of her doctoral studies in my laboratory, was the ideal person for a study of this kind. She managed to form personal relationships with many Holocaust survivors, and thanks to her sensitive approach they agreed to spend several nights in the laboratory so that she could study their dreams. A few of them went so far as to confess that this was the first time since the war that they had agreed to talk about their experiences in the concentration camps. Three groups of volunteers participated in the study: one consisted of Holocaust survivors who had succeeded in adjusting to a new life after the war; the second comprised survivors who had encountered difficulties in their family life, their work, social life, and their health after the war; and the third consisted of native-born Israelis of the same age as the survivors, who had suffered no traumas in the past. Each participant spent five nights in the laboratory for the purpose of reporting on their dreams, and we expected to find great differences in the character of the dreams of each of the three groups.

Therefore, we were extremely surprised when we examined the results. The Holocaust survivors who had adjusted well to life in Israel recalled a mere 33 percent of their dreams, while those who had encountered adjustment difficulties remembered approximately 55 percent of their dreams. The native-born Israelis, as expected, remembered 78 percent. The percentage of forgotten dreams in the well-adjusted group was extremely high. While the native-born Israelis, even when they did not manage to report on a dream after being woken up from REM sleep, nevertheless remembered that they had indeed dreamed, the well-adjusted survivor group vehemently denied any possibility that they had dreamed. This unusual finding is extremely interesting, for such a low percentage of dream reports after a planned awakening from REM sleep had never been recorded in any previous study.

It is important to emphasize that apart from the forgetting of dreams, we found no differences at all between the structure and quality of the sleep of the well-adjusted survivors and that of the native-born Israeli group. The two groups had precisely the same amounts of REM sleep. The sleep of the survivors who had not adjusted well was poor; they had difficulty in falling asleep and were disturbed by frequent awakenings. Analysis of the dream contents reinforced our feelings about the dream process in that it highlighted fundamental differences between the two survivor groups and the native-born Israelis. The few dreams reported by the well-adjusted survivors were short, dealt with trivial, everyday subjects, and were devoid of any display of feelings. The survivors themselves displayed almost total indifference to them after awakening. In contrast, half of the dreams reported by the poorly adjusted survivors reflected anxiety; some of them were real nightmares, often concerning the Holocaust. One of the volunteers, a survivor of Auschwitz, reported the following dream after awakening from REM sleep: "I was standing on the Auschwitz station platform when Dr. Mengele [the Nazi war criminal] suddenly appeared and began sending people to the left, to the crematoria, or to the right, to the forced labor camps. I did not know which way to turn and began to run between the two groups. One of the dogs held by the Gestapo soldiers suddenly jumped on me and was about to bite me. At that moment, you awakened me."

This was an almost true-to-life reconstruction of this particular survivor's arrival at Auschwitz. We concluded that the "erasure" of the well-adjusted survivors' dreams worked in their favor as it prevented the traumatic experiences of their pasts from surfacing and disturbing their sleep. During their sleep, this group adopted the strategy used by numerous survivors during their waking hours over the years: complete avoidance of any discussion whatsoever of their Holocaust experiences. This avoidance was no easy thing. Many survivors experienced guilt and shame at their inability to share their Holocaust experiences with others, even their closest relatives. In many families, this avoidance of any discussion of the past became a painful bone of contention, especially with the younger generation, who refused to reconcile themselves to it. One of the most touching results of the publication of our study was the letters we received from Holocaust survivors thanking us for conducting the study. They said that the findings had in some small way eased their burden of guilt about their inability to discuss what they had been through in the camps. Once it became clear that their successful avoidance of remembering the nightmare of the Holocaust, while awake and asleep, was their way of ensuring their full adjustment to life after the Holocaust, they felt a lot better. On the other hand, survivors who were unable to avoid remembering were less successful in their adjustment. This explanation of the erasure of well-adjusted Holocaust survivors' dreams was not received at all enthusiastically by the more conservative psychiatrists and psychologists, who held that the dream and its interpretation play a central role in the treatment of the post-traumatic patient. The possibility that the erasure of traumatic memories and the repression of dreams might aid the survivors in their adjustment ran contrary to the basic assumptions of the conservative approach.

Yaron Dagan, a clinical psychologist, conducted a study in my laboratory that was similar to that on the erasure of Holocaust survivors' dreams. He studied people who had suffered war-related post-traumatic syndrome as an aftermath of the 1982 war in Lebanon. Unlike the group of healthy volunteers of the same age who remembered the majority of their dreams, the post-traumatic sufferers remembered only about half. As the depth of sleep affects dream recall, we also studied it in these veterans: the findings showed that their sleep was indeed deeper than that of the healthy volunteers. This is one of the possible explanations for the paucity of their dreams. During the study, we discovered that similar findings of "deeper sleep" in post-traumatic casualties of the war in Vietnam had been reported by Milton Kramer, an American sleep researcher who extensively studied dreams in traumatized patients. However, these findings had been shelved because they were inconsistent with everything known at the time about sleep disorders under posttraumatic conditions.


## THE TENNIS DREAM

Eye movements, which are one of the prominent signs of dream sleep, have aroused the curiosity of many researchers. Was the role of eye movements during dream sleep identical to the role they played during wakefulness? Did the eyes follow the action of the dream, or was there no relationship at all between the dream story and eye movements? The simplest and most direct way of studying the meaning of eye movements was to seek a link between the story of the dream and the direction of the eye movements. Recording eyeball movements is done by the application of electrodes above and below, to the right and left of the eyes, thus enabling us to follow both vertical and horizontal eye movements and to test whether they are linked to the action of the dream story. Some studies support the theory of a relationship between the direction of eye movements and the dream story. First, it was found that active dreams which were characterized by numerous events and a high level of activity generated greater eye movement than passive dreams, in which there was a low level of activity. Second, it was found that there are dreams in which the direction of the eye movements can be followed according to what was happening in the dreams at the time of their occurrence.

By far the most convincing example of the relationship between eye movements during REM sleep and the dream story is the "Ping-Pong" dream recorded at the Stanford Sleep Laboratory and described by William Dement in his book *Some Must Watch While Some Must Sleep* (p. 118). Dement gives the example of a series of twenty-six left-to-right, right-to-left eye movements, at the end of which the subject was awakened and asked to report his dream. He recounted that he had been watching a game of Ping-Pong and just before he was awakened he had been following the ball from side to side for a few seconds. A similar case was recorded at the Technion Sleep Laboratory. In one of our studies

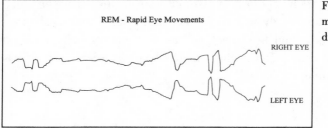

Fig. 22. Rapid eye movements during dream sleep

we noted eye movements which were reminiscent of Dement's Ping-Pong configuration. Although we had not intended to awaken the subject in order to obtain a dream report, we were unable to resist the temptation. We woke him up and asked him what he had been dreaming about. His initial reply was very strange. He had dreamed that he had been playing the guitar with a well-known Israeli pop group. He had been standing on the stage and the show had been about to begin. He described the hall and the other members of the group. At that moment, a heretical thought flashed through my mind: Perhaps, in spite of everything, no relationship existed between eye movements and the dream story? But then the subject went on to tell us that "just before you woke me up, I saw that there was a problem. I didn't understand what was going on, they weren't starting to play, and there I was, looking right and left, again and again, at the other members of the group, waiting for the signal to begin, but it didn't come." The configuration of his eye movements during the last seconds prior to his awakening was consistent with his looking left and right, waiting for the signal to begin playing.

Despite these two convincing examples, it must be pointed out that in the majority of recordings made of eye movements during REM sleep, it is difficult to find any regularity or definite direction. This is not unusual, for even in the eye movement recordings of someone who is awake, it is difficult to pinpoint any regularity except when the subject is watching a clearly defined activity such as a game of tennis or Ping-Pong.

A third proof of the existence of a relationship between eye movements and the dream story can be found in sleep studies of blind subjects. The dreams of the blind, especially those who have been blind from birth and those who lost their sight during their childhood, do not include sights or scenes. Their dreams are characterized by noises, the sense of contact, and emotional experiences. When the sleep of blind people is studied in the sleep laboratory, we find that there are no eye movements during their nonpictorial dream sleep. In a study conducted at the Technion Sleep Laboratory, we found a correlation between the concentration of the eye movements during dream sleep and the number of years the subject had been blind; the longer the subject had been blind, the sparser his or her eye movements.

Two types of eye movement take place during dream sleep: single, isolated movements and groups of movements. Blind people lack the groups of movements, while single movements may be observed during their dream sleep. Our conclusion was therefore that the two types of eye movements during dream sleep possibly fill different roles. Although the movements which appear in groups are indeed related to the dream pictures, the source and function of the single movements have yet to be identified.

One of the assumptions raised about the role filled by the single eye movements linked them to the process of information retrieval from the brain's data storage in order to build the dream story. The link between eye movements and the recall process can be proved by a simple experiment. By observing the eyes of a subject who has been asked a question which requires him to remember a picture—for example, "Whose picture appears on a five-dollar bill?"—we can discern that the recall process is linked to eye movement. The subject moves his eyes as though he were searching for the required information somewhere off in the distance. It is therefore probable that at least some eye movements during dream sleep are linked to the information retrieval process or the processing of that information in order to build the dream.

The findings of two anthropological studies on the REM sleep of primitive tribes support a possible link between eye movements during REM sleep and the processing of information. Two intrepid researchers conducted studies on the sleep configurations of Senegalese and Indonesian native tribes whose lifestyle has remained unchanged for thousands of years. They found that the only difference between the sleep characteristics of Westerners and those of the two tribes was in eye movement structure during REM sleep. Members of both tribes had fewer eye movements during dream sleep. The two researchers, Michel Jouvet and Olga Petre Quadens, a Belgian neurologist, reached the same conclusions—eye movements during dream sleep express, among other things, the processing of information which has been received during the day and is retrieved at night by the dream-creation mechanism. As members of primitive tribes are not exposed to the vast amounts of information and stimuli that modern Westerners experience, their sleep contains very little information processing of this kind. As we shall see, experiments on animals indicate a relationship between physiological "dream" sleep and the processing of information, and the consolidation of traces of memory in the brain.

# 9

# Dreaming as a Separate Reality

I cannot conclude my discussion of dreams without mentioning a subject which is raised almost every time I address an audience. The question is usually preceded by a personal story that runs something like this: "I once dreamed that my brother went on a trip abroad. While he was away he was involved in a road accident in which he sustained head injuries. Two weeks after my dream, it came true in every detail." The teller of the story usually adds more details—for instance, that the car in the dream was identical to the one in the real-life accident.

A further example of this type of personal story is: "I was experiencing a problem at work which bothered me for quite a long time. One morning, I awoke with a complete solution to the problem, which had appeared in my dream." With dreams of this type, the teller usually adds details and color which indicate that the problem had indeed been solved in his dream.

During the course of my lectures I have heard dream stories about death, sickness, finding money, scientific discoveries, planned journeys, marriage, and divorce, all of which, according to the people who recounted the stories, came true or at least provided them with guidance for solving their problem. It would therefore seem that modern civilizations differ little from their ancient Babylonian, Assyrian, Egyptian, or Greek counterparts, which all perceived dreams as a practical means of foretelling the future or providing guidance in their everyday lives. The ancient Egyptians bequeathed us a comprehensive catalog of dreams. Now in the British Museum, the Chester Beatty papyrus, which came from Thebes in Upper Egypt and was written around 1350 B.C., includes some two hundred dreams. A distinction is drawn between good and bad dreams, and the papyrus records the symbols with the help of which the Egyptians interpreted their dreams.

Some well-known oral evidence also indicates that dreams can indeed provide help in solving problems, even scientific ones, and also be an inspiration for artistic creativity. The most famous of these stories is that of the discovery of the benzene ring by the German chemist Friedrich August Kekule von Stradnitz. The molecular structure of benzene was one of the most complex problems faced by organic chemistry in the last century. The structure of organic molecules depended on their physical and chemical characteristics; in all of them, the atoms were united in a straight line. Kekule discovered that the benzene molecule must be represented as a ring; according to him, he made the discovery in a dream. At a scientific congress in 1890, Kekule described his discovery thus (as cited in Gruber's *History of Science* article): ". . . and once again the atoms whirled before me. . . . In my mind's eye, which was filled with countless similar images, I could see large, strange forms and long chains. The forms writhed like snakes. Suddenly, something happened. A snake grasped its own tail and formed a ring-like form which spun before my eyes. I felt as though I had been struck by lightning, and awoke." Kekule summed up his lecture to the congress with the words "Let us learn to dream, gentlemen, and then perhaps we shall learn the truth."

Solutions to scientific problems apart, dreams have also been the source of literary and musical inspiration. Robert Louis Stevenson put his dreams to good use in his writing. When he was young, his dreams were mainly nightmares, but they later gave way to pleasanter dreams of travel and scenic views, and thereafter he began to create entire stories within his dreams. He was also able to continue his dreams from one night to the next. Almost the entire plot of *The Strange Case of Dr. Jekyll and Mr. Hyde* derived from a single dream. Stevenson related, "I had been trying for a long time to write a story about the dualism that exists in every person. It sometimes dominates one's entire thought. . . . For two days I had exerted my brain in an effort to find some kind of a plot. On the second night I saw in my dream: Hyde, hunted because of his crimes, drinking the philtre and becoming Dr. Jekyll before the very eyes of his pursuers. I completed the rest of the plot after I awoke and was fully conscious."

Giuseppe Tartini, the eighteenth-century violinist and composer, related the following story about one of his best-known compositions. He dreamed one night that he had made a pact with the Devil, who undertook to serve him. To ascertain the Devil's musical talents, he gave him a violin and ordered him to play. The Devil then played with such consummate skill that Tartini awoke in a state of high excitement, took up his own instrument and tried to replicate the Devil's playing. Although he did not fully succeed in reaching the heights of the Devil's virtuosity, the dream provided him with the inspiration to compose his most famous work, which he called, not surprisingly, "Trillo del Diavolo" (The Devil's trill).

It is difficult to know how much truth there is in these stories because they are intended by their very nature for the "believers" who use them to promote their own beliefs in dreams. So as the years go by, pieces of information vital for the assessment of whether the matter in question was a real dream or another mental process associated with sleep, are omitted.

At least some of the stories are related not to a dream which occurs during REM sleep but rather to falling-asleep fantasies. Kekule's story, for example, began with a dream that took place after he had laid his head on his desk and tried to nap for a few minutes. As we have no evidence that Kekule suffered from narcolepsy, an illness in which REM sleep appears immediately after the sufferer has fallen asleep, there are no grounds for assuming that his "revelation of the ring" appeared during REM sleep. Even more disappointing to those who believe in solving problems in dreaming are the claims that Kekule stole the idea of the benzene ring from an earlier French researcher. Stevenson's story, too, is questionable, as he suffered from chronic insomnia for years and would spend hours in a state of drowsiness, trying to fall asleep. He claimed that during these efforts to fall asleep he experienced numerous visions, which he described in great detail. It is entirely possible that the characters of Dr. Jekyll and Mr. Hyde appeared before him during one of those long, sleepless nights, and not in a dream. But as we shall soon see in the case of Mr. R., there are people who do dream in a story-like way, and their prolific dreams can easily provide a wealth of plots and stories.

Despite the doubts regarding the veracity of the stories of discoveries through dreams, we cannot ignore the possibility that they may indeed provide assistance in finding solutions to everyday problems and may also become an inspiration for discovery and creativity. If we remember that the raw material of dream stories is those subjects which occupy us during the day, it is possible that they, in new and original forms, may provide the dreamer with fresh viewpoints and perhaps even the solutions to everyday problems. The following examples illustrate this possibility.

A department manager in a large plant had a problem: one of his workers was unsuited to the job he was doing. He mulled over the problem for a long time. What was he to do with the worker? Fire him? Transfer him to another department? If so, to which department? And so on. For reasons that were many and varied, he found it hard to decide, and this disturbed his sleep. He awoke from a dream one morning in the certain knowledge that he had found the solution to his problem. He had dreamed that he had attended a fancy-dress party together with all the staff of his department, including the worker who was the cause of the problem. The problem worker's costume was the hit of the evening and reminded him of the uniform worn by postal workers. On awaking he realized that a job in the plant's mail office would suit that man's talents to a tee! There is no doubt that the dream helped him solve the problem, despite the fact that it was a perfectly ordinary dream. It is probable that if we were to remember even a small fraction of our dreams, we would be astounded to discover to what extent they are built of everyday happenings and to what extent we can find solutions to our problems in them. Nevertheless, I would not recommend waiting for a solution to a problem to present itself in a dream, because you might have to wait for a very long time.

If it were possible to control dream content and scenario, could we then expedite the solving of problems? It appears that the belief in human ability to control the scenarios of dreams exists in many cultures. In his book *The Road to Ixtlan,* the eminent anthropologist Carlos Castaneda meets Don Juan, the old Yaqui Indian sorcerer who teaches the importance of dreaming to the warrior: "A warrior, is a man who seeks power, and one of the avenues to power is *dreaming* . . . although he doesn't call them dreams, he calls them real," says Don Juan. "*Dreaming* is real for a warrior because in it he can act deliberately, he can choose and reject, he can select from a variety of items which lead to power, and then he can manipulate and use them, while in an ordinary dream he cannot act deliberately." Castaneda persists: "Do you mean then, Don Juan, that *dreaming* is real?" "Of course it is real," replies Don Juan. "As real as what we are doing now?" "I can say that it is perhaps more real. In dreaming . . . you can control whatever you want."

It may be assumed that Don Juan's somewhat obscure remarks about the ability to control dreams were taken from ancient Indian mythology. It is no rare occurrence for people to be aware that they are dreaming at the time the dream is actually taking place, and even to intervene voluntarily in the course of the dream. There are also those, albeit few in number, who regularly experience "lucid dreaming," as it is known in the literature, several times a month. Steven Laberge, who completed his doctoral studies at the Stanford Sleep Laboratory, is one of the lucky few to be blessed with this faculty. He was able to draw upon personal experience in the study of the phenomenon in the sleep laboratory.

## LUCID DREAMING

Laberge discovered that the lucid dream indeed occurs during REM sleep and is usually characterized by specific signs of brain activity, such as vigorous alpha wave activity and a high density of eye movements, indicating a high level of arousal. In many cases, the lucid dream occurs when the dream story has frightened or even terrified the dreamer, but the decision that "it is only a dream" doubtless helps to alleviate the fear. Despite the great interest shown in the lucid dream, Laberge encountered some difficulty when he came to publish his laboratory findings in scientific literature. Many people claimed that the high level of arousal indicated that the subject was in a state of half-waking from dream sleep, and not actually dreaming. In order to prove that the subject in question was indeed dreaming, Laberge and his colleagues tested the subject's ability to signal and report on his dream at the very moment it occurred. They found that subjects who tended to dream lucid dreams were indeed able to do this by blinking their eyes during their REM sleep, and moreover that during their lucid dreams subjects were able to perform complex tasks according to directions given to them prior to falling asleep. Performance of tasks during the lucid dream was verified by electrophysiological recordings. For example, when one subject was ordered to move his finger slowly from side to side in front of his eyes, prior to falling asleep, slow eye movements appeared on the electrical recording of the eye muscles during REM sleep. These were identical to eye movements which followed the finger when the subject was wide awake and the hand was truly moved. The subjective experience of the lucid dream in this case was similar to that experienced when the subject was awake. The dreamer was fully aware of the movement of the finger and the entire hand, although in reality, of course, the hand was not moved at all.

As in the enhancement of the remembering of dreams by motivation and suggestion, preliminary evidence shows that the remembering of lucid dreams can be improved. People with strong motivation to dream lucid dreams will increase their chances of doing so. Can the lucid dream be directed to better help us face our daily problems more creatively? Some believe it can. Rosalind Cartwright, one of the most productive dream researchers, used dreaming in a therapeutic technique. She hypothesized that dreamers can recognize a bad dream while still in the process of dreaming, and are able to stop it. Furthermore, by learning how to identify the bad dreams, dreamers can also learn to change the script of the dream into a more positive direction.

## THE STRANGE CASE OF MR. R.

Dream literature contains numerous cases of famous dreamers who documented their nocturnal experiences over many years in dream diaries. Michel Jouvet is a prime example. Another remarkable dreamer was Marquis d'Hervey de Saint Denis, a nineteenth-century French professor of Oriental languages who recorded his dreams from age thirteen and gained Freud's admiration as a result. The marquis, who was a lucid dreamer, had an amazing ability to control his dreams, to be totally aware of them, and to wake up at will in order to record the dream as close as possible to the time of its occurrence.

In recent years at the Technion Sleep Laboratory, we have been witness to another outstanding phenomenon. Mr. R., like Saint Denis, is able to wake up at the conclusion of his dreams and record them accurately. Some of his dreams are extraordinary, for unlike in his regular dreams, Mr. R. himself or people known to him never appear in them. These dreams are complete, logical stories which usually deal with a single subject from start to finish, yet Mr. R. is neither emotionally involved nor plays a role in the plots; he is simply an onlooker. The stories are many and varied; some are richly imaginative and full of humor. A fine example is the dream he had on September 20, 1981, the report of which we quote verbatim:

It is the custom of the Eskimo tribes to send their aged, who have become a burden on the tribe, into exile. In effect, this is the equivalent of a death sentence. A certain Eskimo, who was not that old and who was still active in tribal affairs, suffered from an embarrassing complaint—he was sensitive to the cold— a complaint that in any other society than this would certainly not have been unusual. On a couple of occasions he was caught stealing fish oil from the tribe's storehouse. He asked that the thermostat on the central heating system be raised as high as it would go. The tribe was unable to shoulder the expenditure and they decided to send the cold-sensitive Eskimo to his death in the northern snow fields. Unlike other exiles who waited on one of the icebergs for death to claim them, the Eskimo did his best to survive and began to march away from his tribe. After two days on the march, he met an expedition which was trying to get to the North Pole by dog sled. The members of the expedition were so impressed by the Eskimo's story that they gave him a special electrically heated suit so that he could overcome his sensitivity to cold. Happy with his gift, the Eskimo began to make his way back to the tribe. When he tired, he found a cranny in the snow and fell asleep there. He gave no thought to the heat produced by his fine new suit. The heat melted the ice below him, and he fell into the resulting hole and drowned. When his fellow tribesmen reached the spot, they were unable to fathom how a hole in the shape of a human body had appeared in the ice. How could the water at the bottom be warm? After a great deal of deliberation, they listened to the explanation provided by their chief: their fellow tribesman had drowned as a result of his sins and had gone straight to hell. This did not prevent them from returning to the hole time and again in order to use its hot water to make tea.

Even if this story had been told as one which originated from an awake imagination and not one of sleep, its originality and richness are most impressive.

In other instances, Mr. R.'s dream stories were shorter than the above example; sometimes only short sentences, usually sayings with a moral or catch-phrases like "You can find the best food in Paris on the Boulevard Ravioli [sic]."

When I first read Mr. R.'s dream stories, which had all been dreamed in his mother tongue, German, and translated into English, I doubted whether they could be termed true dreams. Therefore, I suggested that he spend a few nights at the Sleep Laboratory so that we could awaken him from REM sleep and obtain the dream report under controlled conditions. To my great surprise, the results of the laboratory tests verified Mr. R.'s reports. He reported on dreams in thirteen out of fifteen awakenings from REM sleep; nine of the thirteen dreams were normal in that he was the "star" or the roles were filled by people of his acquaintance. Four reports fitted the story-like dream category, and two of them were very similar to stories that he had reported previously.

On one of his awakenings from dream sleep he reported that just before awakening he had seen the following sentence: "Mosquito bites in the United States are more painful than those of the Israeli mosquito because the United States is much bigger than Israel." But the greatest surprise awaited us after the sleep recordings of November 28–29, 1984. Mr. R. awoke from his fifth REM sleep and reported that he did not remember a dream. He muttered one word which he said "was stuck in his mind": the word was "carbide." The sleep technician, who was skilled in interviewing subjects on their awakening from REM sleep, tried to get him to volunteer further information, but in vain. All that Mr. R. was able to report was the one word, carbide. He added that it was "some kind of smelly gas." Carbide does have a particularly pungent smell which can usually be detected after the oxy-acetylene welding of metal. Mr. R. rejected any possibility that he had ever worked in this particular field at any time in his life. He knew what carbide was but could think of no reason why that particular word had appeared in his REM sleep.

Three days after Mr. R.'s sleep test, on December 3, the worst industrial accident in history took place in Bhopal, India. In an explosion at a chemical plant, more than four thousand people lost their lives and a further twenty thousand were injured. The plant was owned by an American company called Union Carbide. I can still remember my shock when I heard the news over the radio. The coincidence was amazing. What is the probability that the name of the company which owned the plant had been mentioned in the dream of a man whose dreams were in any case so strange and unusual? I immediately called Mr. R. to find out whether he too had heard the news, and he had. His initial reaction was, "It's only a coincidence. I don't believe in fortune telling."

Mr. R.'s strange dream was one of those cases which a scientist who wants to protect his good name files away under "impossible observations." I am convinced that if it had happened to anyone other than one of my subjects, I would have found the story hard to believe. And yet it happened just as I have described it, and I feel that the description should remain uninterpreted. I am by no means trying to conclude, or even hint, that the future may be guessed or foretold through dreams. It is almost certain that this was a unique coincidence, but I leave my readers to draw their own conclusions.

To this very day, Mr. R. continues to send us his strange dream reports every few months, and they currently number more than four hundred. As the years have gone by, he has noticed that their frequency has decreased, and these days he wakes up at the conclusion of a dream story only once every few weeks. I have no convincing explanation of the phenomenon, and so it joins the other reports of unusual dreams which have appeared in scientific literature, dreams which provide evidence of the multifaceted character of the abundant world that is created in our brains each night.

# 10

# Do Fish Dream?

One way to understand the importance of sleep is by studying the sleep of species lower on the phylogenetic scale. A comparative study of this kind presents us with a fundamental limitation which is linked to the methods used. The findings of the exciting changes which occur in nervous system activity during the transition from wakefulness to sleep have dictated the use of very clear and rigid definitions of the term *sleep,* and the criteria according to which we can define the transition "between wakefulness and sleep." On the many occasions on which I am asked to provide a scientific definition of sleep, I usually begin by describing the variations in the electrical activity of the brain which occur during this transition, rather than the behavioral changes that accompany falling asleep.

Although it is a simple matter to feign sleep, one cannot fool the electrophysiological recording instruments. And indeed, in some animals, electrical brain activity during sleep resembles that of humans, but in the primitive nervous systems of insects, fish, or even amphibians and reptiles, similar activity cannot be identified. How, then, can we define the sleep of fish or insects without the help of brain wave recordings? Perhaps they do not sleep at all?

Prolonged observations of fish show that, in some cases at least, indisputable and wide variations in activity levels exist during the day-night cycle. There are times at which the fish does not stop moving, while at other times it sinks to the bottom of the aquarium, where it remains almost motionless. If we try to disturb it when it is in the latter state, we find that its response threshold is high. There are even those who claim that the fact that one can grasp the tail of a shark without fear while it is resting at the bottom of an aquarium is the best proof that the shark is asleep. However, I know of no researcher who would take his life in his hands in order to prove this in a controlled experiment!

Insects, fish, amphibians, and reptiles all meet the behavioral criteria of sleep: behavioral quiescence, a stereotypic species-specific posture, elevated arousal threshold, and rapid change in state after intense stimulation.

There is evidence that behavioral sleep exists in bees, wasps, flies, dragonflies, grasshoppers, butterflies, and moths, which all have periods of behavioral quiescence. Furthermore, enforced behavioral wakefulness in cockroaches and scorpions is followed by a compensatory increase in behavioral quiescence that is similar to the increase in sleep time after sleep deprivation. Yet there are no distinct mammalian-like variations in the characteristics of electrical recordings of the nervous system of these species during periods of rest or activity.

In reptiles we find the first signs of electrical brain activity which may be the precursor of the mammals' electroencephalogram. High amplitude and sharp spikes have been recorded in the brain of the caiman during behavioral quiescence. Interestingly, after enforced wakefulness there was an increase in spike activity, suggesting that it may be specific to behavioral sleep, resembling the relationship between the high-amplitude delta brain waves and deep sleep in mammals. Similar high-amplitude spikes were recorded in turtles and tortoises. It should be mentioned, however, that not all researchers agree that these spikes are related to behavioral sleep. Since body temperature decreases in reptiles during this state, some believe that the high-amplitude spikes were caused by the decrease in body temperature.

The majority of researchers who have studied sleep of animals agree that "true sleep"—a change in behavioral state which is also accompanied by characteristic variations in the electrical activity of the brain—first appeared on the evolutionary scale only after the development of the forebrain, and that this, too, was only in warm-blooded animals.

The electrophysiological characteristics of both paradoxical sleep and the other sleep stages are clearly shown in the avian world. As we have no clear evidence which shows that animals do indeed dream, I shall use the term *paradoxical sleep* in this chapter to indicate the sleep stage that is parallel to REM sleep in humans. In chickens, for example, the transition from wakefulness to sleep is accompanied by raised electrical voltage of the brain waves, a slight drop in neck muscle tonus, and a lowered pulse rate. During paradoxical sleep, on the other hand, there is a sharp drop in neck muscle tonus, an acceleration of brain wave frequency, a drop in electrical voltage, and a burst of eye movements. In other birds, there is rarely a drop in the neck tonus. Although the electrophysiological characteristics appear similar, there is a great difference between the cycle of chickens' sleep stages and that of mammals. Although the duration of mammals' paradoxical sleep is measured in minutes, and in humans it can continue for as long as half an hour, this type of sleep in chickens, and birds in general, lasts no longer than ten or fifteen seconds. Therefore, the relative amount of REM sleep in chickens does not constitute more than 3–12 percent of their total sleep, which may amount to only a few minutes every twenty-four hours. Sleep-wakefulness cycles are also different. Many birds do not have long, uninterrupted episodes of sleep but combine short episodes of sleep with open-eye periods characterized by wakefulness-like electrical brain activity, but without changing their specific sleep posture. This has been called "vigilant sleep" because it allows the bird to maintain periodic vigilance while at the same time allowing an unknown sleep process to continue.

Moreover, some birds are often seen to sleep for brief periods with only one eye closed, and for that brief moment it has been suggested that one hemisphere of the brain shows electrical signs of sleep, while the other shows signs of wakefulness. Perhaps this type of one-eyed sleep episode has evolved as an adaptation to the need of migratory birds. The use of radar to follow migrating birds showed that European swifts spend the night in flight. Some believe that they sleep during this time, and it is also possible that sea birds sleep on the wing. Although as yet unproven, perhaps these brief eye openings during sleep aid the bird to maintain its course without deviation and, at the same time, allow the brain to benefit from sleep-related processes.

Vigilant sleep, one-eyed sleep, brief sleep, and the uniqueness of the avian paradoxical sleep are all evidence of the adaptation of sleep to the special living conditions of the organism. In the course of evolutionary development, sleep developed in a manner similar to that of other instincts which evolved in tune with the life styles and living conditions of each species. Birds, which usually roost or perch high up during sleep, may have developed less paradoxical sleep because of their peculiar sleeping conditions. For the same reason, they have no loss of muscle tonus in what little paradoxical sleep they do have. Perching birds simply cannot allow themselves long periods with the slack muscles that characterize paradoxical sleep. It would be interesting to check this hypothesis by investigating paradoxical sleep in the emu, kiwi, and ostrich, all of which sleep outstretched on the ground.

## ANTELOPES AND BEARS: HOW DO THEY SLEEP?

Although the basic characteristics of sleep are identical in almost all mammals, big differences in the duration of sleep, the relative amount of paradoxical sleep, and sleep in other stages still exist between various species. The sleep of more than 150 species has been studied scientifically, and the amount of time each species spends in the various sleep stages has been measured. When the relationship between sleep characteristics and the other characteristics of each of the animals was tested—size, brain weight at birth, gestation period, and so on—it was found that various factors were linked to paradoxical sleep and to sleep that is characterized by slow and synchronized brain waves. Sleep duration was linked to the animal's size: the larger the animal, the shorter the sleep. Irene Tobler of the University of Zurich, the eminent contemporary animal sleep researcher, reported that elephants sleep for only three to six hours a night, of which two hours are spent standing. Like the elephant, the majority of large animals spend a large part of their sleeping time standing, until they reach paradoxical sleep, when they lie down. Why do large animals sleep so little? One possible explanation is related to their food requirements. Large animals need appropriately large amounts of food in order to survive, and this is particularly true of the herbivores that consume food of a low caloric value. As they devote a great deal of their time to foraging for food, the time remaining for sleep is curtailed accordingly. It should be mentioned, however, that large animals also have low metabolic rates compared to those of smaller creatures. It is therefore possible that the length of sleep can be explained by inverse relationship with metabolism rather than by the need to gather food, or other behavioral explanations.

On the other hand, the relative amount of paradoxical sleep was linked to the level of danger to which the animal was exposed in its environment—whether it was prey or predator, hunter or hunted. As a rule, so long as the animal in question has a greater number of natural enemies hunting it, its paradoxical sleep is diminished. The "danger" factor in paradoxical sleep was explained by the elevation of awakening thresholds during paradoxical sleep, which endangers the prey during sleep. However, it should be noted that animals which typically fall victim to predators are not those caught sleeping but those that are more vulnerable to attack, such as the immature, physiologically unfit, or old.

Interestingly, paradoxical sleep varies also with the degree of maturation at birth. In species that are born fairly mature, such as the guinea pig or the sheep, paradoxical sleep at birth is low and near adult level. In species born immature, such as rats, cats, and humans, initial amounts of paradoxical sleep are very large. In kittens, during the first ten days of life paradoxical sleep occupies 90 percent of their time. Therefore, some scientists have suggested that paradoxical sleep is a carryover from fetal life, a form of fetal sleep.

In general, if we compare the way animals sleep with other behavioral characteristics, we will see a clear resemblance. To demonstrate this principle, I shall compare the sleep of a predator, such as the bear, with that of an animal that is usually prey, the antelope. The bear, which fears no enemies in its natural environment, lives at an extremely slow tempo which is in direct contrast to that of the antelope. Bear cubs develop slowly after birth, taking a long time to stand on their own feet and break away from their mother, and the birth itself is bound up with the preparation of a suitable lair. The bear eats and drinks slowly, and the mating of two adult animals may last for hours. In accordance with the bear's life style and behavior, its sleep has become analogous to a sleep that is long and deep. In contrast, the antelope lives in permanent danger and as a consequence is always alert for even the smallest sound. The antelope gives birth extremely rapidly in open ground, without the benefit of prior planning or special preparations, and within seconds of its birth the newborn animal is on its feet and running around. The antelope eats and drinks very quickly, and the mating of two adult animals is over in seconds. The antelope's sleep is brief, frequently interrupted, and lasts for only a few minutes at a time. We still await electrophysiological studies of sleep in the bear and the antelope to verify if the relative amounts of paradoxical sleep and other stages of sleep fit this description.

The best example of the adjustment of an animal's activity-rest rhythm to its life style and environment is undoubtedly hibernation, or winter sleep. This phenomenon is characteristic of many animals that live in the polar regions. During the long winter months, they dig themselves into a protected place and enter a state of dormancy, which for many years was perceived as a particular form of sleep. It is clear today that hibernation is a condition that is totally different from sleeping. In fact, it consists of a drastic reduction in the activity of all the life-supporting physiological systems, in order to minimize energy expenditure as far as possible. This reduction of activity has a high adjustment value, especially during the months in which foraging is made impossible by local climatic conditions. And yet hibernation and sleep are bound up with one another, for hibernation begins during sleep.

## HALF-AWAKE AND HALF-ASLEEP

Sleep studies conducted on animals have revealed that the first appearance of paradoxical sleep apparently took place some 180 million years ago. This is based on the existence of paradoxical sleep in the opossum, a North American marsupial which is thought to be a "living fossil" or survivor of that early period.

So far, there are only two species of mammals in which paradoxical sleep cannot be found in the same form as in other mammals. They are the dolphin, which is considered to be extremely intelligent, and the echidna, one of the three extant egg-laying mammals, a prehistoric evolutionary relic which survived the transition from reptiles. The echidna sleeps for twelve hours a day: its sleep is quiet and characterized by slow waves. (Recent research suggests that the echidna may in fact have paradoxical sleep, but these findings are controversial and the issue remains unresolved.) The sleep of the dolphin is strange, not only because of the absence of paradoxical sleep but also because of its unique brain activity. Nearly all the documented studies on marine mammals have been conducted in Moscow by Prof. Lev Mukhametov and his colleagues, who, after years of experimenting and surmounting numerous technical prob-

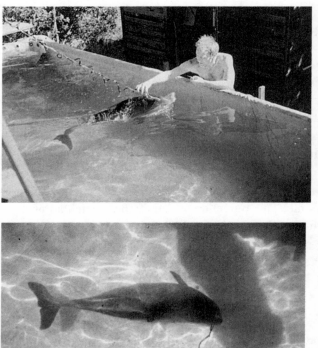

Fig. 23. *Top:* Lev Mukhametov with one of his dolphins. *Bottom:* Sleep recording cable attached to a dolphin in a sleeping position.

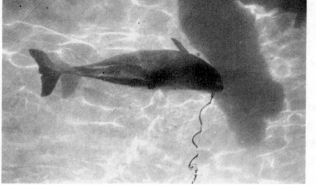

lems, succeeded in recording the electrical activity of a sleeping dolphin's brain. Mukhametov and his team were surprised to find that the dolphin sleeps with only half of its brain while the other half remains totally alert. The electrical activity of the dolphin's brain during sleep is similar to that of land mammals and is characterized by high-voltage, slow brain waves, but this activity always appears in only one hemisphere. At the same time, the electrical activity in the second hemisphere—low-voltage, fast waves—indicates wakefulness. The two hemispheres alternate every one to three hours during sleep: first the left hemisphere sleeps, then the right, but never both at the same time. The duration of sleep in each hemisphere varies and sometimes lasts for two hours or more. During sleep, dolphins kept in aquariums usually swim in circles, in the same direction, as though they were doing so automatically. Prevention of sleep in one hemisphere of the brain is compensated in that hemisphere only and does not change the sleep pattern of the second hemisphere.

Here, too—as in the sleep of birds—we cannot but be surprised at how sleep has adapted itself to the dolphin's unusual physiological requirements. The reason for the dolphin's unihemispheric sleep is the control of its respiratory function. Respiratory activity in mammals is under the control of two brain centers, the voluntary and the automatic, both of which are located in the brain stem. These two centers regulate breathing in order to ensure a regular supply of oxygen and the removal of carbon dioxide. The voluntary center is mainly active during wakefulness, and with its help we are able to stop and renew our breathing as we wish. The center's activation allows human beings the necessary coordination between speech and respiratory activity.

During sleep, the voluntary respiratory center stops functioning and the automatic center takes over. The working of this center is similar in principle to that of the automatic pilot in aircraft, varying as it does the depth and rhythm of breathing in accordance with the level of oxygen and carbon dioxide in the blood. Special sensors measure the levels of gases in the blood unceasingly and transmit the information to the control center, which accelerates or decelerates the breathing rate accordingly, without having to resort to volition. As we shall soon see, one of the most severe, and common, sleep disorders is caused by a dysfunction of the automatic breathing centers during sleep. But unlike humans and other mammals that have a dual system of breathing centers, the dolphin has only one, the voluntary center. In order to ensure the continuous activity of the voluntary center, permanent cerebral arousal is a prerequisite, so the dolphin cannot permit itself the luxury of deep sleep in both cerebral hemispheres at the same time. When Mukhametov and his colleagues administered a sleeping drug to a dolphin, it caused sleep in both hemispheres, and as a result the dolphin experienced difficulty in breathing. The absence of paradoxical sleep in dolphins could perhaps be also explained by the particular conditions under which it lives. As previously mentioned, the dolphin continues to swim in perpetual motion while asleep, and this could be disrupted if paralysis of muscle tonus were to occur, as it does in paradoxical sleep. There is also evidence that uni-hemispherical sleep occurs in other species of marine mammals, like a certain type of seal.

## DO CATS DREAM?

As we have seen, paradoxical sleep is not exclusive to human beings. Apart from the dolphin and echidna, in which it is absent or perhaps takes a different form, it can be clearly identified in all mammals and most birds. Moreover, it is often easier to discern paradoxical sleep in animals like the cat and the dog than in humans. In dogs, for example, paradoxical sleep can even be discerned without the help of electrophysiological recordings. In paradoxical sleep, dogs are more active than humans; they move their legs, ears, and whiskers, wag their tails, and sometimes even seem to bark or whine, so that the observer might easily think that the animal is experiencing something in its sleep.

Does this heightened activity of the dog during paradoxical sleep constitute evidence that it is dreaming? Although we have no direct answer to this question, there is some indirect evidence that paradoxical sleep in animals is indeed related to a dream-like experience similar to that of the human dream. The first controlled, scientific study in which this issue was examined was original in the extreme, but for reasons that remain unclear, it only provided a preliminary report. In order to try to test whether monkeys undergo a dream-like experience during paradoxical sleep, the researchers trained a monkey to pull a handle every time that movies showing images and views were projected onto a screen. Once the animal had mastered this, an electrophysiological recording of its sleep was made so that it could "report" on its dream. The monkey pulled the handle instinctively during paradoxical sleep, as though it were seeing the movies. These observations contained some evidence that the monkey had experienced something that resembled the movies to which it had learned to respond, during paradoxical sleep. I do not know why only a brief summary of this study was published, but it is possible that the preliminary findings were not verified by further observations or that something happened to the monkey during the study and the researchers were forced to abandon it before it was completed. It is no wonder that a study of this kind requires many months of intensive training of the animal before sleep tests can even begin.

Further evidence that animals undergo a dream-like experience similar to that of the human dream was provided by Michel Jouvet's work on cats. The cat, which spends the greater part of the day sleeping and whose sleep comprises a high percentage of paradoxical sleep, is almost certainly the "champion dreamer."

By means of some extremely precise surgery, Jouvet succeeded in severing the neural pathways along which the nerve impulses that inhibit the spinal motor nerve cells are transmitted during paradoxical sleep. As a result of the surgery, the cat was able to enter paradoxical sleep without a loss of muscle tonus, and then an amazing phenomenon was observed: as the cat entered paradoxical sleep, it stood up and embarked upon the most complex behavioral repertoire, which bore no relationship to what was happening around it. After observing numerous cats, Jouvet concluded that certain behavioral patterns which appear in paradoxical sleep after the removal of the inhibitor always recur, including attack, defense, and exploration. To anyone watching, it would appear that the animal was attacking invisible enemies inside its cage; it arched its back, its hackles rose, and it growled threateningly. A few seconds later it backed away in panic, as if it sensed an unseen attacker. There were some cases in which the cat rose and began sniffing around the cage as though inspecting it for the very first time. Attempts to divert the attention of the animal with flashes of light while it was involved in its dream, or even by tempting it with food, met with no response. The cat's behavior was completely automatic; some considered it to be reminiscent of human sleepwalking. Sleepwalkers too, usually children and teenagers, behave automatically without responding to their environment. Sleepwalking, however, does not occur during paradoxical sleep but always in the deep sleep of stages 3 and 4, and therefore it cannot be explained by the removal of the mechanism which inhibits muscle tonus.

Jouvet's findings in cats, which were later substantiated at Adrian Morrison's laboratory in Philadelphia, show intensive nervous activity in the motor cerebral cortex during paradoxical sleep. The motor paralysis which occurs during paradoxical sleep provides a defense for the sleeping organism. If inhibition did not occur, what would prevent the activation

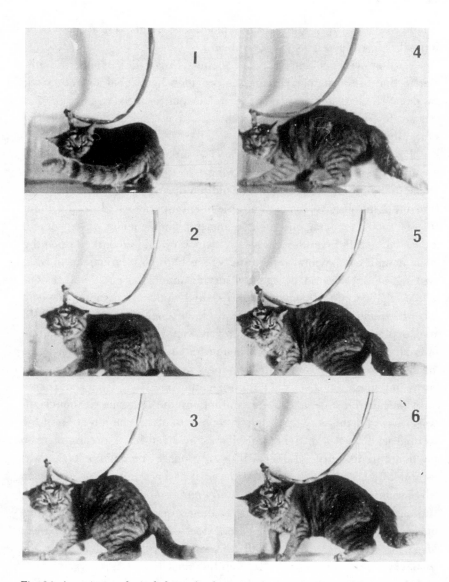

Fig. 24. A cat in paradoxical sleep after lesioning the muscle tonus inhibitory mechanism. The cat stands up, arches its back, and raises its hackles in order to scare off imaginary enemies.

of the behavioral pattern which is created completely automatically in the cerebral cortex? The importance of the defense mechanism is highlighted here, because the greatest dangers that lie in wait for sleepwalking children are injuries caused by bumping into a variety of objects, tripping, and falling.

In recent years, scientists have observed human behavioral patterns reminiscent of the strange behavior of Jouvet's cats. The first to describe this phenomenon were Carlos Schenk, Mark Mahowald, and their colleagues from Minneapolis, who reported on people, predominantly males, who came to the sleep laboratory complaining of violent behavior while they were asleep. According to the evidence furnished by their bedpartners, they would wake up during the night and begin to act extremely violently for no apparent reason, smashing anything that was in their way. At a scientific conference on sleep, Schenk presented a videotape documenting one such "violent awakening." It was not difficult to be impressed by the extraordinary force of the subject's violent behavior and by the fact that it was completely "automatic." Recordings made of people who suffered attacks of anger and violence during sleep showed that they occurred after brief awakenings from REM sleep. Although the reason for this disruption of dream sleep mechanisms is not fully understood, there were in some cases indications of brain degeneration.

What is the reason for intense activity in the motor cerebral cortex during paradoxical sleep? Jouvet, impressed by the orderly motor behavior of his brainstem-lesioned cats, hypothesized that one of the roles of paradoxical sleep was to train the neural networks which are related to instinctive behavior. Instincts are an innate form of behavior—in other words, patterns of motor behavior which are not learned but stamped on the nervous system even before birth. The behavioral patterns of numerous species which involve attack, defense, or copulation are instinctive, and the animal performs these actions from birth, without being trained to do so. The human's first smile which lights up the face during REM sleep is another instinctive pattern of behavior; the perfect "dream smile" appears in infants without training or learning. Jouvet speculated that during paradoxical sleep these neural networks are activated independently of the muscles which are linked to the nerve cells and inhibited by the brain stem. This activation is similar to a trial run of a giant computer program conducted to ascertain that the computer is in working order before it is put to practical use. This "running-in" period allows the programmer to uncover any unforeseen problems and improve the computer's various functions before it goes on line. According to Jouvet, because of the decisive importance of the instincts to the survival of the species, the neural networks linked to instincts are checked every night.

As we shall see, this is only one of many theories about the role of paradoxical sleep which have been propounded in recent years.

# 11

# The Need for Sleep

Some people come to the sleep laboratory asking for help with their sleep disorders, bitterly complaining that they "haven't slept a wink, not even for a moment, for months and perhaps even years." Many sufferers from sleeplessness are convinced that they have not slept at all for many days on end, but not a single person suffering from total sleeplessness for more than a couple of days has yet been found. It is, in fact, possible to go without food longer than going without sleep.

Sleep is indisputably a basic need, but its duration varies, often considerably, from person to person. In one of his treatises, Rabbi Moses ben Maimon, or Maimonides, claimed that we have to sleep for one-third of the day, or eight hours. The happy inhabitants of Sir Thomas More's Utopia also slept for precisely eight hours. These myths are apparently the source of the magic number of hours that human beings are supposed to have to sleep.

At the Technion in 1980, we conducted a survey of the sleeping habits of fifteen hundred manual workers. We found that the average Israeli industrial worker sleeps not 8 hours but approximately 6.5 hours during the week, and almost 8 hours at weekends. High school pupils do not sleep more. In a recent survey of some sixty-five hundred schoolchildren, we found that a quarter of high school teenagers sleep no more than 6 hours each night. It is not surprising, therefore, that three quarters of them regularly nap during the day. Can we conclude from our study that teenagers and manual workers have too little sleep? Can we link sleeping time with productivity or work accidents, or achievements in school in teenagers? As I shall discuss shortly, in some cases we certainly can.

The shortest sleep documented in professional literature is that of Miss M., a seventy-year-old retired district nurse from

London, who slept for about an hour every day. While the study was being conducted, she expressed great surprise when the technicians who ran the laboratory tests had to be relieved in order to catch up on their sleep! She was unable to understand people who slept for long periods and "wasted so much time." Ray Meddis and his colleagues who reported this unusual case admitted that "we are very much at a loss to explain why Miss M. should be as she is."

Another phenomenon, which was never studied in a laboratory, was a man who could make do with even less sleep than that cited in the above case. In 1974, the first international congress of sleep researchers from all over the world took place in Edinburgh. On their way to the congress, several researchers visited a certain London orphanage, the director of which had gained prominence after his appearance in a BBC television film showing that he slept for a total of fifteen minutes a day. The researchers had wanted to see this wonder for themselves, for the orphanage director had shattered every known theory about the number of hours a human being needed to sleep. He had also opened a window on the possibility that sleep was not a necessity at all and that we could perhaps live without it. I was fortunate enough to be among those visiting the orphanage, and indeed I found that the director was a most impressive gentleman. I called on him at 11 P.M. and found him playing with a group of some fifty children. Everyone there was prepared to swear that "the director never sleeps," and the impression I received was that he did not sleep for more than a few minutes every day. He told me that when he had served as a wing commander in the Royal Air Force, his comrades had exploited his extraordinary sleeping habits to the full and had appointed him permanent night duty officer!

When I tried to tempt him to come to Israel for tests in our sleep laboratory, he almost threw me out. It appeared that every sleep researcher who had visited him had made more or less the same proposal. He told me quite simply: "I am not a rat or a guinea pig to be moved from laboratory to laboratory and have my sleep studied. You can believe me or not, but this is the way I am and this is how I sleep."

But these are the exceptions, representing the most extreme "short" end of the sleep duration continuum. Today there is a consensus among researchers from different countries that sleep need, like most biological traits, is normally distributed. This takes the form of a bell-shaped figure ranging from about 4.5 to 10.5 hours, with an average between 6.5 and 8.5 hours. The middle grouping includes about 65 percent of adults.

Several researchers have attempted to determine if there are differences in personality types between short and long sleepers. Ernest Hartmann, an American psychiatrist, has devoted a great deal of time and effort to this subject. He compared people who slept for an average of 5 hours a night with people who slept for 9 hours or more.

Hartmann reported that short- and long-sleeping individuals were of different personality types. The people who slept for the shorter period were efficient, energetic, and active, they derived a great deal of satisfaction from their work and lives, and were not disposed to complain. The subjects who slept for longer periods were less homogeneous. Some were the "eternal student" type who spent most of their lives at university moving from course to course; some could be defined as devout nonconformists, and these tended to question and complain about the experiment, the political and economic situation, and so on.

Can we assume then that the length of sleep is responsible for the differences of personality which exist between long- and short-sleepers? Or perhaps it is the other way around and efficient, energetic people who are always busy and "never stop working" sleep less because they see sleep as "a waste of time." Which is the chicken and which is the egg? Unfortunately, Hartmann's findings were not shared by other investigators.

Bernie Webb, who also examined the relationships between personality profiles and hours of sleep, concluded that they are completely unrelated. He summed up his disappointing findings in *Sleep, the Gentle Tyrant:* "It seems that just as there are people with large and small ears, so there are naturally long and naturally short sleepers. Such differences may have little influence on (or be the results of) other traits such as differences in ear size or hair color." In any case, it is no surprise to find that extremely short sleepers have different life styles and habits than extremely long sleepers. After all, people who sleep only 5 hours a night must find ways to fill their extended waking hours.

Examining the lives of some famous historical personalities does not clarify the picture. There is absolutely no conformity here: genius inventors and distinguished soldiers belonged to either one of the two extremes, long sleepers or short sleepers. Both the inventor of the light bulb, Thomas Alva Edison, and Napoleon Bonaparte were short-sleepers; Edison viewed sleeping as a waste of time and went so far as to say that people who spent a great deal of time sleeping were fools. We can assume that had he known Albert Einstein he would have changed his mind, for Einstein belonged to the long-sleeping category.


## REDUCING SLEEPING TIME

Another question that bothers a great many people is, How many hours does a person need to sleep in order to function properly? Unfortunately, there is no unequivocal answer. We should not be alarmed by a baby who sleeps too little; if the infant is alert and happy during its waking hours, then it is getting sufficient sleep. A person who sleeps for 5 or 6 hours a night, is alert and energetic during the day, and does not feel either chronic fatigue or a strong desire to sleep, is almost certainly not in need of additional sleep.

A further question is, Can a person who is used to sleeping a certain number of hours every night change his sleeping habits? This issue becomes critical in a country like Israel, where military service is obligatory. Thus, high school students, having completed their final examinations, get used to sleeping until lunchtime. Then they join the army, where they usually sleep about 6 hours a night and have to rise between 5 and 6 A.M. Some claim that they are absolutely unable to adapt to army life simply because they have to get up so early. How far, then, can sleeping habits be changed or reorganized?

The possibility of reducing sleeping time appears very attractive. If such a reduction could be accomplished without ill effects, then we could add more time to our working life. Jim Horne, a British sleep researcher, divided sleep into two types: "core" or indispensable sleep, and "luxury" sleep. According to Horne, the organism needs only sleep which is vital and which is composed mainly of deep sleep, while the remainder may be classed as a luxury and can be reduced without causing any harm. This phenomenon is analogous to eating, says Horne. Although it is true that food is vital to the existence of the organism, we do not eat simply to exist but for a variety of reasons and in amounts which exceed the body's requirements.

Surprisingly, the effects of the chronic limitations of sleep time have attracted less attention than total sleep deprivation, although they are more common in everyday life. Few have attempted to examine what happens when sleep time is reduced by, say, 20–30 percent for an extended period of time. Bernie Webb and Bob Agnew investigated the effects of reducing young adults' sleep time from 7.5–8 to 5.5 hours for sixty days. They found that in spite of the reduction in sleep time—which mostly affected REM sleep that was only 25 percent of baseline values—there were no major behavioral consequences. In their *Psychophysiology* article, they concluded: "A few hours of transient or even chronic sleep loss of a relatively extended period resulting from work requirements, personality disorders or insomnia, are not likely per se to result in major behavioral consequences."

For obvious reasons, the United States Navy has also studied this subject extensively. Three people who were used to sleeping 8 hours a night were chosen to participate in the navy's first experiment. They were assured of payment if, over a period of four to five months, they could reduce their sleep quota by thirty minutes every three weeks. The researchers wanted to find the lowest limit at which the subjects would "break" and to see how the gradual cutback of sleep affected their behavior. The volunteers were given the option of leaving the study once they had reached the lower limit of their sleeping hours. A further objective, which was concealed from the subjects, was to examine whether they would maintain the change in their sleeping habits after the payments had stopped.

All the subjects cut their sleeping hours during the navy's experiment; one reached 4 hours of sleep and the other two got down to 5 hours. The price paid during the final stages of the experiment was high: all the subjects showed significant signs of lack of sleep, and were tired and irritable. Yet the most surprising result of the experiment was that eight months after its completion, and after the subjects had been paid, all three participants who had previously been used to sleeping 8 hours a night reported that they had cut 1 or 1.5 hours from their daily quota of sleep. When the subjects were questioned about the change, it appeared that they had learned to make do with less sleep and thus profited from additional hours of wakefulness.

In the wake of these findings, the U.S. Navy group at San Diego conducted another experiment on five married couples who were students at the University of California at San Diego and who were used to sleeping 7.5–8 hours a night. This time, the subjects were given different adaptation periods; the first half-hour reduction, from 8 to 7.5 hours, was made within ten days and the second within three weeks. Once the subjects had reached less than 6 hours sleep a night, they were allowed a month in which to adapt to every additional thirty-minute reduction. As in the first experiment, it was found that all the couples reached less than 6 hours of sleep a night; one couple reached 5 hours a night, and one even managed to reach 4.5 hours.

The irritability and tiredness which had been observed in the first experiment became evident during the final stages of the second. A few couples were unable to stand the strain and were forced to sleep for at least an hour during the day, but a year after the conclusion of the experiment not one of the subjects had returned to his or her previous sleeping habits. The "big winner" was a man who maintained 5.5 hours of sleep a night instead of 8 and who claimed that he felt fine, was functioning well, and that he now felt that he had been wasting 2.5 hours every day on unnecessary sleep. When we multiply this reduction by the number of days in a month, the number of months in a year, and finally by the number of years of the subject's life expectancy, his "profit" was indeed immense.

Is it so? Can we actually safely cut down sleeping time and "earn" precious waking time? Studies conducted during the last few years have refuted this simplistic notion. Persons who cut down their sleep pay a price in the form of increased sleepiness during the day, even though they may explicitly deny any ill effect. Sleepiness is a subtle sensation; the increased awareness of sleep disorders associated with excessive daytime sleepiness (see chapter 19) has shown us that many people live their day-by-day lives literally half-asleep, without being aware of it or even ready to admit it. I have met scores of patients who vehemently denied being sleepy and, were it not for the tenacity of their spouses, would never have arrived at a sleep clinic for consultation. It is always amazing to witness a heated quarrel between couples on the subject of excessive sleepiness: while one stubbornly denies it, the other recalls the exact time and place where the spouse dozed off. There is no doubt that persons who sleep too little, and consider sleep a waste of time, can go on with their lives if sufficiently motivated.

Denial of sleepiness is no longer accepted as a testimony of adequate alertness. Using the multiple sleep latency test described in Chapter 5, Mary Carskadon has shown that restricting sleep time to 5 hours for seven consecutive nights caused a profound effect on daytime sleep tendencies during the last two days. In half of her subjects the level of sleepiness was considered "pathological"—that is, they reached the same level of sleepiness as that of patients suffering from sleep disorders. The rest of the subjects reached "borderline" levels of sleepiness. For the entire group, the latency to fall asleep during the day was halved from 14.3 minutes at the start of the study to 7 minutes after seven nights of sleep restriction.

Adi Gonen, a doctoral student in my laboratory, utilized one such technique to investigate the change in sleepiness observed in young adults after being drafted to the army. He objectively determined sleepiness levels in high school graduates when they slept 8.5–10 hours a night, and then again three months after they started a military training course which allowed them to sleep 6 hours, according to army regulations. Adi observed a profound increase in sleepiness in every one of his subjects. Since the course did not involve intensive physical activity, the increased sleepiness must be attributed to the decreased sleep time.

The above observations led to the conclusion that many people, particularly young adults, suffer from chronic sleep debt. Actually, this was noted twenty years ago by Webb and Agnew, long before the issue of excessive sleepiness and its price became fashionable among sleep researchers. Many of us who sleep late on weekends, or nap during the day whenever possible, are not enjoying luxurious sleep but just attempting to keep our sleep accounts balanced.

## "ACROBAT'S LEAP": EIGHTY HOURS WITHOUT SLEEP

There have been many studies in recent years aimed at examining the effects of reduced sleeping hours or the complete deprivation of sleep on behavior and functioning. Experiments on human sleep deprivation usually last two to three days, or four at the most. After scrutinizing the results of these studies, it is quite surprising to find that total sleep deprivation over several nights does not cause dramatic changes in either the subject's behavior or physical condition. The results of these studies indicate a certain drop in daily functional levels, which is shown by lethargic reactions and speed of thought. It was found that subjects asked to perform complex tasks demanding a high attention level and a heavy memory load were more prone to failure than when asked to complete simple tasks which were performed automatically. Changes of mood were also observed; depression and an increased feeling of tension and heightened interpersonal sensitivity. Sleep-deprived people tend to withdraw within themselves and to respond aggressively to trivial matters. It may be said that so long as the hours and days without sleep increase, so does the feeling of fatigue and drowsiness. These feelings also change according to the time of day. The most difficult time in sleep deprivation experiments is the early hours of the morning, which, it will be remembered, is the time when body temperature and the alertness level are at their lowest. Those conducting the experiment have to use all their powers and energy to keep their subjects awake at this time, for the desire to sleep is so great that sleep forces itself upon the subjects in many and varied ways. A nocturnal stroll in order to help combat drooping eyelids may appear to be the solution, but it poses a problem when we come to analyze the findings of the study. It becomes difficult to differentiate: Were the changes observed in the subjects' behavior the result of sleep deprivation only, or were they also affected by the increased and continuous motor activity needed to keep them awake?

One of the phenomena which drew a great deal of attention was the appearance of hallucinations and distorted perception. Although they affected only a small number of subjects, they were both dramatic and the cause of some anxiety among the experimenters. In one experiment I witnessed, the objective was to examine the effects of more than 80 hours of sleep deprivation on the functional ability of soldiers under combat conditions. The sixty-four young soldiers who had volunteered for the experiment were determined to complete their mission successfully. They wanted to prove to their officers and to the large group of psychologists and doctors who were with them throughout the experiment that their functional levels would not be affected. The first night and the following day passed without incident. The soldiers' morale was high and they showed almost no signs of nodding off or involuntary falling asleep. This picture changed radically during the second night, and even more on the third. In the course of these nights, and particularly in the early hours of the morning before the sun came up, the experimenters had to maintain a permanent watch on the soldiers to make sure that they did not fall asleep. Some fell asleep while standing, sitting, and even walking. I met a group of the soldiers for a talk at 2 A.M. on the third night of the experiment. They rocked from side to side in an effort to stay awake while standing. The exhaustion was evident in their voices when they answered my questions; their speech was slow and came with a great effort. During that same talk, a few of the soldiers reported that in the last few hours they had begun to talk to themselves or to various objects that they had encountered which they imagined to be human beings, and this had both confused and frightened them. One soldier related a weird experience that he had undergone a few minutes before our meeting. While marching together with his comrades, he had suddenly seen himself marching in front of himself. He said that it was as though he had been split into two different people, with one watching the other!

A number of researchers have reported on this phenomenon of distorted perception and hallucinations under conditions of prolonged sleep deprivation. Someone has called it "sleep deprivation psychosis" and claimed that prolonged sleep deprivation may cause serious mental disturbances, but it must be emphasized that the phenomenon is not as common as some people think. It occurs in only a small number of people and once the low point of the night passes, it disappears without trace. Indeed, the soldiers' behavior changed beyond recognition after the sun had come up. On the fourth day of the experiment, after more than 80 hours without sleep, the soldiers completed their military tasks with the same degree of skill and speed as they had when the experiment began and they were fresh after seven hours of sleep. At the conclusion of the experiment, which for some of the participants had continued for more 80 hours, they slept for a mere 8–10 hours. As numerous researchers have reported, sleep after an extended period of wakefulness is different from regular sleep, particularly in the voltage of the slow brain waves.

On the face of it, the findings of the military experiment on sleep deprivation (which was given the apt code name "Acrobat's Leap") proved that military missions can still be executed at a high level of skill even after four days without sleep. But this came as no great surprise to the veterans of previous wars. The ability to continue functioning without sleep over a period of days during combat is well known. Under these conditions it should be remembered that motivation is incredibly high and that anxiety, stress, and physical activity all help to fight off sleepiness. The upper limit of continuous activity without sleep under conditions in which energy reserves are exploited totally appears to be approximately four days.

## SLEEP DEPRIVATION IN THE RECORD BOOKS

Two efforts to stay awake for more than 200 hours have become part of the lore of modern sleep research. In 1959, a radio broadcaster called Peter Trip tried to remain awake for 200 hours to raise money for the American March of Dimes. He settled into a completely transparent broadcasting booth placed in New York's Times Square, where passersby could see him throughout his marathon. Only toward the end did he begin to show signs of behavioral deterioration when, during the night, clear signs of psychosis accompanied by hallucinations appeared. Trip began to suspect that people were drugging his food in order to make him fall asleep. William Dement, who related Peter Trip's story in *Some Must Watch While Some Must Sleep,* said of himself that sometimes, when he had to stay on for long periods at Nathaniel Kleitman's laboratory, he would suddenly find himself distrusting his companions and suspecting that they were plotting against him. As a sleep researcher who was fully aware of the delusive effects of lack of sleep, he would tell himself: "There is no reason to feel this way. I know that it's ridiculous and I know that the cause of the delusions is lack of sleep." Yet the irrational fears and the complete awareness of their source occurred simultaneously.

The second attempt to set a record for staying awake was scientifically documented. In 1965 Randy Gardner, a seventeen-year-old from San Diego, challenged the record of 260 hours which appeared in the *Guinness Book of Records.* As Randy's attempt progressed, public and scientific interest heightened. After 70 hours, Dement's Stanford team joined television camera crews and reporters as observers. As expected,

Randy had most difficulty in staying awake at night, when he needed a superhuman effort to overcome the attacks of compulsive sleepiness. Dement, who followed the experiment closely in order to make completely certain that Randy was not sleeping, related that one of his most impressive memories of the experiment was a game of basketball he played with Randy at 3 A.M. on the last night. Randy beat him, and Dement claimed that the young man's victory showed that his motor and physical functions had not been impaired. After setting a new record of 264 hours, Randy held a press conference and answered the questions put to him with a great sense of humor. When the conference was over, Randy went to sleep in the U.S. Navy's San Diego sleep laboratory, where he slept for 10 hours and 40 minutes. When he woke up, he felt refreshed and energetic all day, and slept for only 8 hours the next night, which was his usual quota. Throughout the experiment, no anomalous phenomena such as hallucinations, perceptual illusions, or extreme changes of mood were observed.

The conclusion that can be drawn from the results of Acrobat's Leap and Randy Gardner's feat is that people who are absolutely determined are able to continue without sleep for several days, especially when they have the support of constant monitoring and excitatory stimuli. As the only way to fight off sleep is through energetic physical activity during the critical period of the early hours of the morning, physical fitness is very important. Fit people are simply better equipped to withstand prolonged periods without sleep.

## THE BURNING-LIGHT CULTURE

The Acrobat's Leap experiment began on a Sunday and lasted until Wednesday morning, after more than 80 hours of sleep deprivation. Those who took part in it tended to think that sleep was perhaps not as important to military activities as the sleep researchers claimed. Was it possible to function for a number of days without sleep without any difficulty?

This belief is, in fact, deeply rooted in many military cultures throughout the world. The military glossary in Israel contains the term *burning-light culture,* which defines the common practice of holding staff meetings long into the early hours of the morning and the almost compulsive need of officers to go to sleep long after the last of their men. The light burning in the brigade or battalion commander's room has long since become a symbol of diligence and industry. Not one of his subordinates will dare to go to bed while the commanding officer's light is still burning.

No sooner had I arrived home after Acrobat's Leap than I received a call from a doctor friend who was on a senior officers' course at the time. It was very strange. There I was, still covered with desert dust after a week in the Negev and still very much affected by the experiment and its results. And there was Dr. V. on the other end of the line asking for my help in an urgent matter concerning sleep hours on an army course. At first I was sure that he had heard about Acrobat's Leap and that this was his humorous way of expressing his admiration for the experiment, but it turned out that he had a real problem. The participants of the course he was on were suffering from chronic sleep deficiency. According to Dr. V., they had slept only two to three hours a night for the past two weeks; the men were falling asleep during lectures and exercises and even in high-risk situations like driving. When they had complained to the officer commanding the course, his laconic reply was: "I don't sleep for more than two hours a night either; if I can do it, so can you."

The assumption that everyone needs the same amount of sleep is completely without foundation. Someone who needs six hours of sleep a night will not be able to function well for an extended period on two to three hours, or even five hours of sleep a night. In a situation such as this, the immediate danger is the appearance of compulsive falling asleep during the day, especially during periods of inactivity, though frequently during activity too. Some of these sleep spells are very brief, lasting only a few seconds, but they pose a high safety risk. While driving, for example, it only takes two or three seconds of dozing off to take the vehicle off the road and into a ditch! I suggested to Dr. V. that he go to see his commanding officer again and request a discussion on sleep as part of the course, with the participation of specialists on the subject, and I expressed my readiness to take part. I do not know whether my proposal was accepted or not, but the fact that Dr. V. did not get back to me was evidence enough that there had been an improvement in his sleep hours.

There is no doubt that people who suffer from chronic sleep deficiency do not function well. They are sleepy and tend toward irritability and depression. Israel Defense Forces standing orders state that soldiers should be allowed at least six hours sleep a night, and moreover that they should be compensated in sleep hours after night operations or exercises. Officers, especially of lower ranks, must be taught that prolonged sleep deficiency is not conducive to either heroism or better soldiers.

Insistence on a proper amount of sleep does not apply only to the military. The subject of a recent public debate was the sleeping hours of those employed in professions that contain an element of danger to the public, like drivers, pilots, and doctors. A driver who suffers from chronic sleep deficiency is likely to cause a road accident, not only because of falling asleep momentarily but also as a result of lack of attention and slow reactions in a dangerous situation. There is, therefore, a great deal of logic in legislation that sets out the sleep hours of public-service vehicle drivers and the limitations placed on the number of hours spent at the wheel.

It is somewhat surprising that medicine is the only profession in which the workers are required to carry on functioning regardless of their sleep hours. After a night on duty, interns are required to carry on working throughout the next day, irrespective of fatigue and as though they had enjoyed a full night's sleep. In a Technion Sleep Laboratory study, we found that interns on night duty in the emergency room of a big hospital slept for an average of only 2.5 hours a night. After their night duty stint, they carried on working next day for 8 hours or more without any thought about sleep deficiency, and as most of the interns did at least two night duties a week, we come to an unavoidable conclusion: interns suffer from chronic sleep deficiency, which may severely impair their functioning as doctors. In the light of evidence that the long nights spent on duty by hospital doctors do indeed affect their ability to function normally during the day, public and professional criticism of these work procedures has increased in recent years. The first place in which the work regulations pertaining to doctors have been changed, and their work hours after night duty limited, is the state of New York. The change came about in the wake of a tragedy in which alleged neglect in the treatment of an eighteen-year-old patient (Libby Zion) during the small hours of the night caused her death. The patient's father, a lawyer and journalist, embarked on an uncompromising public crusade to have doctors' work hours changed—and his efforts were crowned with success. From July 1, 1989, residents' work hours in the state of New York were limited to

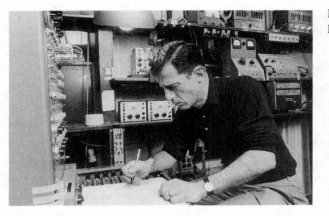

Fig. 25. Allan
Rechtschaffen

80 hours weekly. Since then, many other hospitals have voluntarily changed their residents' working schedules, but no other state has as yet followed New York's legislation.


## THE ROLE OF SLEEP

The findings of the first studies on total sleep deprivation in puppies, which were conducted at the end of the last century, were dramatic in the extreme. After some seven or ten days without sleep, the animals died, but the cause of death was unknown. A postmortem examination showed no change in brain tissue or other vital organs which might have shed some light on the cause of death.

The relatively sparse findings on the effects of sleep deprivation in humans stand in apparent contradiction to those of Henri Pieron from the end of the last century, which proved that depriving animals of sleep for eight to ten days caused their deaths. What, then, is the importance of sleep?

In recent years, great progress has been made in understanding the importance and role of sleep. This progress is the fruit of the research conducted by one of the veterans of sleep research, Allan Rechtschaffen, and his associates at the University of Chicago, where REM sleep was discovered by Aserinsky and Kleitman. As previously mentioned, one of the most difficult methodological problems encountered in every study of sleep deprivation is that of separating the effect of the sleep deprivation itself from that of the physical activity required to stay awake, for the only way to prevent sleep during the small hours of the night is to engage in energetic physical activity. Therefore, when sleep deprivation studies were conducted on animals, the animals were usually made to continue their motor activity in order to prevent sleep. Rechtschaffen had a brilliant idea about how to study the effects of "net" sleep deprivation, which would exclude the unwanted effects of induced motor activity on the laboratory animals. By using a computer, the configuration of the brain waves characteristic of sleep and wakefulness is easily discerned. Rechtschaffen and his associates built an apparatus consisting of a 46-centimeter-diameter turntable divided by a partition. The turntable was mounted on a spindle and placed over a shallow tray of water 2–3 centimeters deep. Two rats, into whose brains electrodes linking them to the computer had been implanted, were placed on the turntable, one on either side of the partition.

The sleep deprivation experiment was conducted as follows: one rat was assigned the role of the test animal while the other was the control; when the computer identified the characteristic signs of sleep in the configuration of the experimental rat's brain waves, it activated the turntable, which began to revolve at a slow speed, wakening the rat and forcing it to walk in the opposite direction to the disk rotation to avoid being swept into the water. If the rat did not wake up, it was carried into the water, which awakened it immediately. The control animal on the other side of the partition received similar treatment, because it was on the same turntable. However, while sleep was severely reduced in the experimental rat, the control rat could sleep whenever the experimental rat was spontaneously awake and the turntable remained still. Thus Rechtschaffen succeeded in depriving the test animal of sleep for many days, while the control animals either did not lose sleep at all or lost it to a much lesser extent. As both animals were subjected to exactly the same treatment, it could be assumed that the stimulation of both was identical, except for the effect of sleep deprivation. According to Rechtschaffen's findings, only the test animals died after two to three weeks without sleep. As with Pieron's findings in his puppies, no severe abnormalities which might have hinted at the cause of death were found in the brain tissue or major internal organs. The main changes observed in

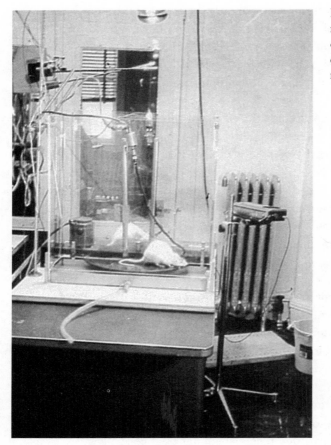

Fig. 26. The apparatus used in the experiments on the effect of sleep deprivation in rats

the test animals were in their fur and general appearance. When I visited Rechtschaffen's laboratory, he gave me a tour of the entire facility. In every corner there was an experimental apparatus and on it, two rats. One glance was enough to tell me which of them was the test animal and which was the control. The test animals' fur was thin, wispy, and befouled even though the animals had not stopped cleaning themselves.

Rechtschaffen and his colleagues' search for the cause of death in their experimental rats could fit the plot of an Agatha Christie thriller. At first they suspected that hypothermia, or drop in body temperature, was the cause, because all experimental rats showed a decline in body temperature. When the experimental rats were kept warm with electric heaters, however, they died nevertheless. Thus hypothermia was not necessarily the cause of death. Breakdown of bodily tissues by accelerated metabolism, as well as systemic infections, was also ruled out by a series of elaborate experiments.

Even though the direct causes of death of the sleep-deprived rats remained a mystery, Rechtschaffen's studies provided new information about the possible functions of sleep. One of the consistent observations was that the test animals increased the amount of food they consumed, while at the same time losing weight. These changes suggest that the sleep-deprived rats have an increased metabolic rate, as though they had an increased need of energy. In fact, near death, the sleep-deprived animals showed energy expenditure which was two to three times higher than the normal rates. What could cause the elevated need for energy in sleep-deprived rats? It could be caused by either excessive loss of heat or a change in the set point of the brain thermostat. In an ingenious experiment, Rechtschaffen's lab showed that indeed the set point of the brain mechanism that keeps internal heat at a constant level was increased by sleep deprivation. They removed the test animal which had gone without sleep for at least two weeks and tested the function of the brain center which regulates temperature. To do this, they used a "heat corridor"—a one-meter-long receptacle, one side of which was heated to 60°C (140°F), while the other was at the freezing point. When a rat which had not been subjected to prolonged sleep deprivation was placed in the center of the receptacle, and the direction it took was studied, it chose to remain and sleep in the area with a temperature of 30°C (86°F). When a sleep-deprived rat was placed in the heat corridor, it chose to remain in the area where the ambient temperature was 50°C (122°F)! The control animals fled from this area as fast as their legs would carry them. The brain centers which control internal thermostats had been altered so that the rats now preferred to be at higher temperatures.

Rechtschaffen and his colleagues concluded that sleep deprivation disrupted the activity of the brain cells responsible for "temperature regulation." In further experiments, when Rechtschaffen prevented only paradoxical sleep, it became clear that paradoxical sleep deprivation did not cause a change in the brain thermostat but was the cause of the disruption in heat conservation. The test animals were unable to keep their body temperature stable and suffered from excessive heat loss.

Interestingly, when sleep-deprived animals were near death and were removed from the turntable and allowed to sleep, all these changes could be reversed while the animals showed large rebounds of paradoxical sleep. On the first day after they were allowed to sleep without interruption, paradoxical sleep was five to ten times greater than normal. Rechtschaffen concluded in 1989 that "the need for paradoxical sleep may exceed the need for other sleep stages when paradoxical sleep loss has been severe or prolonged, or when survival is at stake."

These findings shed new light on the role of sleep, at least in rats and possibly in other small mammals. It appears, therefore, that sleep is vital to the regulation and stability of the organism's internal environment. The complex mechanisms which maintain this stability need sleep, much as far simpler mechanisms in electronic and mechanical systems need periodic servicing. Without sleep, the system loses its equilibrium and this may cause death. Further studies should tell how much of Rechtschaffen's findings can be applied to humans.

# 12

# The Eccentricity
# of REM Sleep

As I have described earlier, REM sleep is characterized by an apparently impossible combination of physiological changes: the disappearance of muscle tonus, the appearance of brain waves which indicate wakefulness during sleep, rapid eye movements, frequent changes in respiration and pulse rates, and the appearance of penile erections in males. Studies employing sensitive techniques which tested energy consumption in the brain and the flow of cerebral blood during sleep revealed that REM sleep resembles wakefulness more than it does sleep, even according to these parameters.

Indeed, the eccentricity of REM sleep does not end there. When the activity of the autonomic nervous system was tested during REM sleep, an astonishing fact was revealed: there is a retrogression in the brain's control levels over the most vital physiological processes. In order to maintain life processes, the maintenance of body temperature and blood gases level at optimal values is of cardinal importance. In Chapter 11 we saw that damage to the mechanisms which control the regulation of body temperature under conditions of prolonged sleep deprivation can cause death. When the regulatory mechanisms of both body temperature and blood gases levels were tested, it was found that they had been functioning normally in every sleep stage except for REM, or paradoxical sleep.

Testing the normal functioning of the regulatory mechanisms is performed thus: A subject goes to sleep in an air-conditioned room and the room temperature is raised or lowered during the various sleep stages; during sleep stages other than REM sleep, the subject's physiological response to room temperature changes is similar to the response of a subject who is awake. If the temperature is raised, the subject will begin to perspire and the capillaries in his skin will expand in order to speed up heat evaporation. All this will take place during sleep, the course of which will not be affected. When the room temperature is raised during REM sleep, no change will occur in the functioning of the temperature regulation mechanisms. If the room temperature is raised gradually even more, the subject will awaken at a certain critical temperature, and only after he has awakened will the body temperature regulatory systems begin to work. If, instead of heating the room, we cool it, we will observe a similar reaction. In sleep stages 2, 3, and 4, physiological changes, the function of which is to preserve body temperature, will occur in the subject. He will begin to shiver, his hair will stand on end, and his capillaries will contract in an effort to reduce heat loss as much as possible. All of these changes will occur during sleep and without the subject waking up. They will not occur during REM sleep unless the subject wakes up beforehand. During REM sleep, the thermostats in the brain—the same nerve cells that sense changes in temperature—will be cut off and therefore will not transmit information to the body temperature regulator mechanisms.

A similar "cut-off" occurs in the nerve cells which "measure" blood gas levels. In order to test the function of the respiratory control system during sleep, subjects were ventilated with a mixture of gases in which the relative concentration of carbon dioxide had been altered. When the concentration of carbon dioxide was increased during sleep other than REM sleep, the respiratory response was identical to that which occurs during wakefulness: the respiratory rate increased and breathing became progressively deeper. In contrast, no change in breathing occurred during REM sleep until the moment of awakening.

The changes which occur in the control of the regulating processes of the internal environment during REM sleep, together with the changes mentioned earlier, reinforce the view that REM sleep is an unusual existential condition that is totally different from wakefulness and sleep stages 1 through 4.

What is the significance of these changes? How can they be explained? When the brain consumes large amounts of energy and the blood supply to it increases, is it then completely cut off from the external and internal sensory organs?

Is it possible that all the brain's energy is invested in such vital processes during REM sleep that evolution has allowed the existence of a situation wherein the organism relinquishes the regulation of its internal environment for short periods?

What would happen if REM sleep were to be prevented selectively? Could we continue to function without it?


## SELECTIVE PREVENTION OF REM SLEEP

That the beginning and the end of REM sleep can be identified with extraordinary precision is an extremely valuable tool for researchers. We can try to learn something of the importance of REM sleep by its selective prevention, and it is a relatively simple thing to create REM sleep deprivation in the laboratory. The subject's sleep must be checked and recorded, and every time the technician sees brain waves and eye movements which typify REM sleep on the electrophysiological recording, he awakens the subject, keeps him awake for five to ten minutes, and then allows him to go back to sleep. He then repeats the process at the following REM period, thus depriving the subject of the best part of his REM sleep. The subject will still enjoy a little REM sleep because the technician needs at least one minute to identify it before he wakes him, and indeed, instead of a hundred minutes of undisturbed REM sleep, he will enjoy only several minutes of it. We must, of course, ensure that the subject is unable to dupe the experimenter by catching up on his lost REM sleep during the day.

All the studies on REM sleep deprivation have yielded two important results. First, the number of awakenings required to prevent REM sleep increases as the duration of the deprivation is prolonged. If on the first night a small number of awakenings is needed—say, an average of ten to twenty—this will have increased to sixty by the third night of the experiment. The reason is that the pressure for REM sleep has been increased. As soon as the subjects close their eyes and try to fall asleep, they enter REM sleep without delay. It is very difficult to conduct an experiment on REM sleep deprivation in humans for longer than five consecutive nights because after the fifth night the subjects enter REM sleep as soon as they fall asleep and consequently have to be woken up again.

William Dement, who carried out the first experiment on REM sleep deprivation in humans, described the reason for terminating the experiment in an article in *Science* magazine: "We had to stop the experiment because there was no way we could awaken the subject and disturb his REM sleep, although we could have stopped his eye movements for short periods. We sat him up in bed and shouted in his ear and at the moment we stopped, his rapid eye movements reappeared immediately. The only way to stop the dreaming was to drag him out of bed and forcibly walk him around the room until he woke up and then keep him awake." In a situation such as this, a night-long struggle ensues between the experimenter, who is responsible for the experiment and who wakes the subject up in order to prevent him entering REM sleep, and the subject, who is doing everything in his power to do just that. Then, of course, the experiment loses its value because what is happening is the prevention not only of REM sleep but of any kind of sleep whatsoever.

The second result of REM sleep deprivation studies also leads to the conclusion that there is a biological need for REM sleep. When the subjects are allowed to sleep undisturbed at the end of the deprivation period, they compensate themselves for the REM sleep of which they were deprived. The first REM sleep will appear earlier, some 40 minutes after falling asleep and sometimes even after only 20 minutes. They will enjoy approximately 150 minutes of REM sleep instead of the "standard" 100.

## THE EFFECTS OF PREVENTION OF REM SLEEP

Dement carried out his experiment in a most original way. As the experiment demanded almost nonstop monitoring of the subjects, he rented a large apartment in New York and moved in with his whole family. One of the bedrooms was set aside for the subjects and the recording equipment was set up in the bathroom. Thus he was able to monitor his subjects day and night and to awaken them every time they entered REM sleep. In this way he managed to prevent his subjects from entering REM sleep for five or six consecutive nights, and one subject even managed to go for seven nights without REM sleep. The principal finding of this experiment was the indisputable proof that human beings need REM sleep, and this was borne out by the subjects' increasing pressure to enter REM sleep.

Dement's experiment gained tremendous acclaim because of one particular observation, which unfortunately was later shown to be marginal and nonrepresentative. One of the subjects suddenly expressed a desire to go to a night club, read pornographic literature, and showed a prurient interest in sex, all of which he had never done before. Dement described the subject in detail in an article in which he claimed that the prevention of REM sleep was liable to cause a radical personality change. In light of the great interest shown in dreams and their place in Freudian theory, this finding provided some kind of incontrovertible proof that dreams were indeed necessary for the preservation of mental equilibrium and that their prevention could upset that equilibrium. But numerous attempts to substantiate Dement's findings failed. The results of many studies of personality changes resulting from REM sleep deficiency in humans varied from nebulous change, expressed in distrust and extreme irascibility, to a dramatic improvement in the mental state of depressive patients. Nevertheless, I still encounter teachers who use Dement's case to convince their students of the importance of REM sleep.

When I was studying for my bachelor's degree in psychology, Dement's articles on sleep were the first ones I read, and they were my principal stimulus for spending many sleepless nights in the laboratory. Their style was spellbinding and it was obvious that they had been written by someone who identified totally with his chosen field. For this reason, Dement's unusual "home" study came as no surprise. But he was not unique: the pioneers of sleep research who were active in the sixties and seventies were mainly psychologists and psychiatrists who, as the years went by, became a tightly knit family. They were all imbued with a sense of urgency in their work. The discovery of REM sleep may be compared to the discovery of a previously unknown continent: wherever you look, new and unfamiliar vistas are spread before you. Each new sleep laboratory experiment held the promise of exciting findings which were yours and yours alone. This feeling of exploring terra incognita is addictive.

The circumstances of my first meeting with Dement reveal a great deal about his character. I was engaged in my doctoral studies at the University of Florida in 1972. I was sitting in my office in the laboratory, racking my brains over the data from the experiment I had conducted the

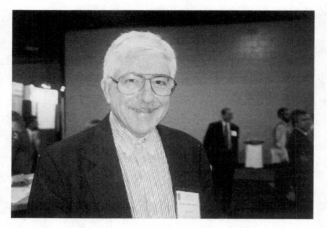

Fig. 27. William
Dement

previous night, when the door opened and a man I did not recognize came in. Two features made a deep impression on me: his thick mustache and his shock of flowing hair. He asked me where Professor Bernie Webb was and apologized for not informing the professor of his visit beforehand, as he was just vacationing in Florida. Webb had just left for Europe on one of his frequent lecture tours. The visitor was disappointed and as he turned to leave, he said, "Please give him regards from Bill Dement."

It should not be difficult to imagine my excitement; there I was, a doctoral student at the beginning of his studies, face to face with the man behind the enthralling articles that had guided me toward spending so many nights in the sleep laboratory. Before I could allow myself to change my mind, I said, "Professor Dement, would you care to have a look at the results of my experiment?" Without hesitation, he pulled up a chair and sat down beside me, and I quickly found myself in an enthusiastic discussion with the high priest of sleep research about the effects on perceptual tasks of awakenings from REM and deep sleep.

Some fifteen minutes later, Dement suddenly grasped his head in his hands—he had remembered that his wife was waiting outside in the car and that he had promised her that he was "just going to say hello to Bernie!"

Many years later, when I reminded Dement of our chance meeting, he could not understand why I had been so excited or why I had viewed our meeting as being out of the ordinary, for he perceived anything connected to REM sleep as a subject worthy of discussion and conversation, even with a young student.

## REM SLEEP AND CEREBRAL AROUSAL

As I mentioned earlier, the selective prevention of REM sleep often has a therapeutic effect on depressive patients. The first to report on this was Gerald Vogel, a psychiatrist from Georgia and one of Allan Rechtschaffen's students. Vogel showed that when patients with endogenous depression were deprived of REM sleep for one or two nights, there was a spontaneous improvement in their mental state. Sleep disturbances, too, disappeared. The depression sometimes passed completely, sometimes the patients' condition was only improved; there was an increase in their activity and their mood improved. When the sleep of depressive patients was tested in the sleep laboratory with the help of electrophysiological recordings, it became clear that it differed from that of normal people. Their sleep contains a very small amount of stage 3 and 4 deep sleep and their REM sleep appears earlier, some twenty to forty minutes after falling asleep compared to eighty to ninety minutes with normal people. The duration of the first REM sleep is longer than that of normal people; it is much more turbulent and is characterized by a great many eye movements which are the primary sign of REM sleep. This is further proof that eye movements during dream sleep do not necessarily only reflect the "dream story."

Why, then, does the prevention of REM sleep improve the condition of the depressive patient? To answer that question, we must first discuss the findings of studies on the prevention of dream sleep in animals.

The technique used to prevent REM sleep with animals is simple and even original. A rat's paradoxical sleep can be prevented by using what is called the "inverted plant pot" technique. It will be remembered that REM sleep is characterized by a sharp reduction of muscle tonus, including that of the neck muscles. An inverted plant pot 7 to 10 centimeters in diameter is placed in the center of a receptacle containing water and the rat is placed upon it. The water level almost reaches the lip of the pot. Because of the pot's small diameter, the rat is forced to keep its head above the water level by using its neck muscles. It is able to hold its head up when awake if its neck muscle tonus is functioning normally, and it can do the same thing during sleep other than paradoxical sleep because, although its muscle tension during this sleep is low, it is still existent. When the rat moves into paradoxical sleep, it is unable to hold its head up, its head touches the water, and it wakes up. Thus, paradoxical sleep in rats can be prevented for extremely long periods, much longer than in humans. In the experiments I described in Chapter 11, Rechtschaffen discovered that selective prevention of paradoxical sleep in rats caused death forty to sixty days after the beginning of the experiment.

What about prevention of paradoxical sleep for shorter periods of time? In these cases there is evidence that the prevention of paradoxical sleep in animals like mice or rats caused increased cerebral arousal. This phenomenon can be tested in a number of ways. One is to examine the effect of paradoxical sleep deprivation on the convulsion threshold using electric shock. When a strong electric shock is administered to the head of a rat, the animal enters a condition of motor convulsions similar to that of an epilepsy sufferer. The convulsion threshold is measured by the strength of the shock required to cause the paroxysm, and it is lowered considerably in an animal with paradoxical sleep deprivation. We can therefore use a much weaker shock to cause the paroxysm in an animal that is suffering paradoxical sleep deprivation than we can after normal sleep, or a deprivation of sleep other than paradoxical sleep. Furthermore, the paradoxical sleep compensation showed by rats after a period of deprivation can be decreased by administering a number of shocks during the deprivation period. The electric shock supplies a kind of substitute for the paradoxical sleep of which the animal has been deprived.

Experiments conducted on cats also verify the existence of a relationship between paradoxical sleep and arousal. Dement and his colleagues prevented paradoxical sleep in cats by awakening the test animals each time they entered paradoxical sleep. After a number of days, the animals' sexual behavior became exaggerated and they began to eat uncontrollably, consuming much more than they had eaten prior to the experiment and than control animals that had undergone prevention of other sleep stages. Dement found that the prevention of paradoxical sleep in cats caused the arousal of the sexual and nutritional instinctive systems. It will be remembered that Michel Jouvet had already shown that detachment of the mechanism that inhibits the skeletal muscles caused cats in paradoxical sleep to exhibit an entire repertoire of behavior that was mainly instinctive. It is therefore probable that the prevention of paradoxical sleep in which training of the neural networks related to instincts has taken place caused an overactivation of the "brain execution" program of nutritional and sexual behavior.

In the light of these findings on the relationship between paradoxical sleep and cerebral arousal levels, we can understand the therapeutic effect of the prevention of REM sleep on depressive patients. These people suffer from a lowered cerebral arousal level and diminished impulses, and any increase in arousal will improve their condition. It should not come as a surprise, therefore, that one of the most efficacious treatments of depression is the electric shock. As we have seen, electric shocks given during the period of paradoxical sleep deprivation decrease the amount of REM compensation later on.

## REM SLEEP AND MEMORY TRACES

Additional evidence linking REM sleep and cerebral arousal has come from studies in which the relationship between memory and REM sleep was investigated. Although there is no precise explanation of the biochemical processes that take place in the brain and which are the substructure of memory storage and retrieval, much research on the way in which information is stored in the nervous system has been accumulated over recent years. In general terms, we can differentiate between at least two types of memory, short-term and long-term. Short-term memory is the first memory storage and is usually limited to between five and nine items, which are retained for no more than thirty seconds. If we do not rehearse the items, they are forgotten. In contrast, the long-term memory storage, the "central information bank," houses items of information which have been acquired throughout our life; from childhood, school lessons, everyday life, visual and auditory information, or motor skills such as riding a bicycle or swimming. After it has been processed, classified, and catalogued, each item is stored in the brain. The way information is stored in the brain is extremely complex, and it appears that each type of information has a specific storage area of its own.

Research conducted in the last few years has shown that the consolidation of memory traces in the long-term memory storage is associated with a period of intense neural activity in certain parts of the brain, of which the most researched is the hippocampus, and with subsequent biochemical processes and structural molecular changes in various parts of the brain. Several studies have indicated a possibility that the consolidation of memory traces for at least certain types of learning occurs during REM sleep. Some studies show that selective prevention of paradoxical, or REM, sleep impairs memory consolidation and subsequently learning; others show that paradoxical sleep increases during the process of successful learning.

Many of the latter group of studies were carried out by the French researchers Elizabeth Hennevin, Vincent Bloch, and Pierre Leconte. Their general procedure was as follows: Prior to the experiment, they carefully monitored their test animals for several days to determine their basal amounts of paradoxical and nonparadoxical sleep. Afterwards, learning sessions were planned in order to record subsequent sleep at precisely the same time of the day as before. In this manner, the researchers showed that paradoxical sleep increased in mice and rats after a variety of learning procedures. For instance, in "active avoidance conditioning," rats learn that whenever a flash of light or a buzzing sound appears, they have to escape to a certain area of their cage to avoid an electric shock. While the rats were learning this task, the researchers found a significant augmentation in the amount of paradoxical sleep during the three-hour recording period after each daily period of training. When learning was completed and the test animals performed the task with almost no mistakes, paradoxical sleep returned to prelearning level. Control animals that were exposed to the same electric shocks and flashing lights or buzzing sounds, but without learning, did not show this augmentation. Similar results were found when the test animals learned to press a lever in order to receive water, or when they learned their way through a complicated maze. When sleep was delayed for three hours after the learning sessions, however, the acquisition of learning was impaired and there was no augmentation in paradoxical sleep. Bloch, Hennevin, and Leconte summarized their studies thus: "It would appear that one of the essential elements for memory fixation is the presence of paradoxical sleep in sufficient quantity, occurring quickly after learning."

Complementary evidence of the importance of paradoxical sleep to learning was provided by the selective prevention of paradoxical sleep. This was conducted in the following way: Rats were trained in a specific test, and immediately afterwards paradoxical sleep was prevented using the "inverted plant pot" technique. After two to three hours, they were removed from the plant pots and returned to their cages. When the animals were tested twenty-four hours later, they showed deficient retention in comparison with control rats that were returned to their cages immediately after the training, or were put on the inverted plant pot for the same time period after spending two hours undisturbed in their cages. Chester Pearlman and Ramon Greenberg, who conducted one of the first REM deprivation studies, concluded that REM sleep occurring immediately after the training was essential for the consolidation of the memory traces in the brain. The observation that the animals in which the prevention of paradoxical sleep was delayed for two hours after the training showed no impairment suggested that memory consolidation in the brain occurred during the first two hours after the training.

Further proof that the damage caused by prevention of paradoxical sleep occurred at a critical stage of memory consolidation was provided by a study in which the electric shock was used very imaginatively. Administering an intensive electric shock to rats immediately after they have learned to perform a certain task causes the "erasure" of what has been learned, but only on condition that the shock is administered immediately after the conclusion of the learning process. The shock has no effect if it is administered two to three hours after the learning because it has no effect on the long-term memory storages but only on the process of memory consolidation. If the claim that prevention of paradoxical sleep impairs the process of memory consolidation is correct, then one would expect that the effect of electric shock on animals after three hours of paradoxical sleep deprivation would be greater than that on control animals whose paradoxical sleep had not been prevented. And indeed, that is what happened. The prevention of paradoxical sleep, at the end of which an electric shock was administered, completely erased any memory traces.

In other studies it was found that the relationship between memory consolidation and paradoxical sleep was far more complex. Learning some tasks was affected by the prevention of paradoxical sleep, while learning others was not. Fulfilling a task of great importance to survival was not affected by the prevention of paradoxical sleep. For example, if an electric shock was administered to a rat at a certain place inside its cage, then from that moment on the rat would identify that place as "dangerous" and would flee whenever it was returned there. This task was not affected by the prevention of paradoxical sleep, because identification of dangerous locations in the animal's natural environment is vital to its ability to survive.

Perhaps for this reason, experiments which were conducted in order to test whether REM sleep was linked to memory consolidation in humans usually yielded negative results. It is probable that REM sleep is necessary in humans only for certain types of learning and remembering. Some findings indicate that REM sleep in humans does indeed play a role in special learning tasks. Consider, for example, sufferers from aphasia, people who as a result of brain damage have forgotten part of their vocabulary. When the language learning process of aphasiacs was observed, it was found that the patients who succeeded in relearning a large part of the words they had forgotten were those whose REM sleep had become extended during the learning period, while the REM sleep of those who failed to relearn their lost vocabulary remained unchanged. It has even recently been found that intensive learning of a new language by young people is bound up with an increase in REM sleep. These findings bring to mind those of Leconte, Hennevin, and Bloch on the increase in paradoxical sleep during the learning period of their mice and rats. Further evidence of a relationship between REM sleep and intellectual aptitude has been reported from experiments on children suffering from mental retardation. The duration of REM sleep in these children is usually shorter than that in normal children of the same age, and it is characterized by fewer rapid eye movements.

Recently, the possibility that only some types of learning in humans are connected with REM sleep has been supported by a carefully controlled laboratory study. A team led by Avi Karni and Dov Sagi, of the Weizmann Institute of Science in Israel, trained volunteers rapidly to recognize the orientation of symbols hidden in images flashed at a very high speed at the periphery of their vision. This particular type of learning is unique because it shows a marked improvement approximately eight to ten hours following a training period. Volunteers who were trained in the perceptual task and then retired to sleep showed the anticipated improvement the following day. Likewise, improvement was found in volunteers who were repeatedly awakened from sleep stages other than REM sleep. In marked contrast, volunteers whose REM sleep was prevented did not show the expected improvement. The researchers proposed that the consolidation of the learning process of this perceptual task occurred mainly during REM sleep. Thus, it is possible that REM sleep is particularly important for procedural types of learning in which humans acquire motor and perceptual skills. Since during the few first months of life infants are busy acquiring new motor and perceptual skills, these findings may also explain the abundance of REM sleep at that particular time in our life.

Despite the relative paucity of findings from studies on the relationship between memory and REM sleep in humans, recent years have yielded some theoretical assumptions which received acclaim. The most popular theory was that of Francis Crick, J. D. Watson's collaborator in the discovery that the sequence of bases in DNA was the genetic code, and winner, with Watson, of the Nobel Prize for medicine. In 1983, Crick and his mathematician colleague Graeme Mitchison published an article on REM sleep in the journal *Nature,* in which Crick and Watson had published their historic article on the structure of DNA some years earlier. Crick and Mitchison claimed that the role of REM sleep was to organize the brain's memories. According to their theory, the brain's memory storage can be compared to tremendous networks of nerves which create innumerable junctions, at each of which interrelated items of information are stored. During REM sleep, the information networks are organized; nonvital items of information that have inadvertently been collected during the day are "erased" from the network. Without this process of nocturnal erasure, said Crick and Mitchison, the vast amounts of information which reach the brain every day would be likely to "jam" the memory banks. They claimed that dreams which take place during REM sleep are composed of those items destined for removal from the memory banks.

I shall not go into the details of how the screening of the memory banks takes place during REM sleep, because this would demand a knowledge of the mathematics specially developed for the new field of "neural network theory," but at the end of their article, Crick and Mitchison categorically stated that the prevention of REM sleep in humans for long periods would cause serious cognitive disruption, similar to that characteristic of schizophrenics. According to them, the experiments in selective prevention of REM sleep in humans were not sufficiently prolonged as to have caused real changes in the cognitive and memory processes of the subjects involved. Was this indeed so?

## Y. H.: A MAN WITHOUT REM SLEEP

About a month after the publication of Crick and Mitchison's speculative article, my colleagues and I published an article in *Neurology*, the journal of the American Academy of Neurology. The subject was the extraordinary findings of an experiment conducted on a young man whose sleep had been monitored at the Technion Sleep Laboratory. The article threw down the gauntlet before all those who had championed the absolute necessity of REM sleep for humans.

Y. H. had been referred to the Technion Sleep Laboratory because he had been awakening in panic while shouting loudly. This particular disorder could have been the result of nightmares during REM sleep or of a disorder, not viewed as pathological, the source of which is in deep sleep and which is usually peculiar to children. It sometimes bothers adults too, but mainly in stress situations. Y. H. was an Israel Defense Forces veteran who had sustained brain injuries from Egyptian shrapnel during the "War of Attrition" on the banks of the Suez Canal during the early seventies. He was confined to a wheelchair and suffered from difficulty in the use of his hands and in his speech. The objective of our tests was to ascertain the source of his panic-stricken awakening. On July 1, 1982, Y. H. was tested for the first time at the Technion Sleep Laboratory, and we found no trace of REM sleep on that first night.

The complete absence of REM sleep from a laboratory sleep recording is extremely rare. It sometimes characterizes patients who are undergoing treatment with a high dosage of antidepressants or sleeping drugs, or those who are under the influence of hard drugs. Y. H. was neither taking medication nor did he suffer from depression, and when he awoke, he reported that he had slept well and normally. In light of the unusual observation, we decided to do an additional recording, but this, too, revealed no traces of REM sleep. Apart from the absence of REM sleep, the sleep recording was perfectly normal.

When I told Y. H. about the results of the second sleep test, he was not unduly upset. His spontaneous reaction was, "OK, I don't have REM sleep, so what?" I remember trying to bring the awesomeness of this medical sensation home to him. I told him that if he really did not have REM sleep, it would be something like a cardiologist trying to listen to the heartbeat of a patient sitting in his office and discovering that he didn't have one! The analogy made Y. H. burst out laughing, but then he agreed, in a sporting spirit and with a certain sense of pioneering, to spend a further six nights in the Sleep Laboratory. We decided to do a complete brain scan using computerized imaging, and also a recording of the electrical activity in the brain stem in order to ascertain the precise location of the shrapnel lodged in his brain. The laboratory findings clearly showed that Y. H. had almost no REM sleep. Although we found some traces of REM sleep on a few nights, on each occasion the amount did not exceed 2–5 percent of his total sleep, while in healthy people of the same age the amount reaches 20–25 percent. Moreover, after analyzing the results of the eight nights of the tests, we found that Y. H.'s sleep was very short. He slept for only 4.5–5 hours but showed no signs of lack of sleep throughout the day.

But the biggest surprise of all was yet to come: The computerized brain scan showed that, apart from the shell splinters that were lodged in the left hemisphere of the cerebrum and in the cerebellum, there was an additional splinter, the existence of which had been unknown, lodged in Y. H.'s brain. This splinter was located in the pons of the brain stem, in exactly the same place that Jouvet, after his work on cats in the seventies, had placed the brain mechanism which controls the activation of REM sleep (see Chapter 13). This was incontrovertible proof that the location of the REM sleep mechanism in humans was identical to that in other animals.

The publication of the case of Y. H. in scientific literature elicited a flood of correspondence, the main thrust of which was the significance of the findings and their ramifications on the numerous theories about REM sleep. That the article was published at almost the same time as Crick's and Mitchison's article on the importance of REM sleep in organizing the human memory system probably contributed to increased interest in the subject. Many wanted to know whether Y. H. had suffered any disruption of his memory or thought processes, but Y. H. had a wonderful memory. Immediately after sustaining his injuries, he had completed his high school studies and had been accepted to law school, from which he had been graduated successfully. Because of the difficulties he had in using his hands, he had relied mainly on his memory during his studies.

In 1984, I spent a sabbatical at Allan Hobson's laboratory in the Department of Psychiatry at Harvard. Hobson, a psychiatrist and neurophysiologist, and his colleague Bob McCarley had developed a mathematical model based on their neurophysiological work which explained the alternation between REM sleep and other stages of sleep. They, too, succeeded in rocking the psychiatric community on its heels with an article in which they claimed that the dream was nothing but a manifestation of cerebral activity that was similar to that of dementia patients.

That year marked the thirtieth anniversary of the discovery of the structure of DNA, and Francis Crick had been invited to give the keynote lecture in Boston to celebrate the historic event. As Crick had been assisted in the preparation of his lecture on the importance of REM sleep by Allan Hobson, he was more than happy to give Hobson's group a "private" seminar on his ideas about the importance of REM sleep. After he had presented his arguments regarding the proofs of the importance of REM sleep in screening the memory systems, and claimed that a person without REM sleep would have to show clear signs of thought disturbance, I presented the case of Y. H., which had been published that month. The case clearly surprised Crick very much; his first reaction was doubt. Perhaps our observations on Y. H.'s memory ability and his thought processes had not been perceptive enough. Could he possibly be suffering from mild disturbances that we had not detected? When I stood my ground and said that Y. H. had no cognitive disturbances and that his memory and thinking were superlative, Crick replied, "Well, this is the exception that does not necessarily prove the rule. Perhaps we should wait for a few years in order to examine the effects of REM sleep deficiency." Indeed, four years later I received a letter from Crick in which he inquired whether I was still keeping a check on Y. H. and whether any change had occurred in his condition. As Y. H. and I had remained friends and continued to meet every few years, I knew that he had become a very successful lawyer. I also knew that in recent years he had become an expert at solving cryptic crosswords, making quite a name for himself in this field, and this certainly did not quite fit in with "thought and memory disturbances."

In order to satisfy Crick's—and to a certain extent my own—curiosity, I called Y. H. and asked him to make a further contribution to science in the form of a few more nights at the Sleep Laboratory. Happily, he agreed without hesitation. In 1988, we conducted a further series of tests on Y. H. which lasted for five nights. The results were identical to those from the tests conducted six years earlier. On three of the nights we found no trace of REM sleep, while on the other two we found only a few isolated minutes. Four years later, Y. H. contacted the laboratory on his own initiative when he was once again troubled by sudden awakenings accompanied by loud shouts. And just as we had found ten years earlier, these were night terrors characteristic of deep sleep. We did not find REM sleep during any of the three nights of recording.

The case of Y. H. is, without doubt, both instructive and confusing. It is instructive because it imposes clear limits on any generalization we may force upon laboratory studies of animals and humans, and confusing because it compels us to ponder the wisdom of nature. Why, over a period of 150–200 million years, did evolution develop such a strange form of existence if we can do very well without it? Could the role played by REM sleep be less vital than we tend to believe? Perhaps it is simply a "fossilized" relic of brain activity that was necessary in the early stages of our development, somewhere in the transition from cold-blooded reptiles to birds and mammals?


## REM SLEEP: A SLEEP FOR ALL SEASONS?

At one of the scientific congresses on the importance of REM sleep, William Dement, whom we met earlier, declared with no little frustration: "If it is indeed true that REM sleep plays no vital adaptive role, then we come to the unavoidable conclusion that REM sleep is one of evolution's most grandiose mistakes."

What, then, is the point of preserving REM sleep, when the sleeping organism is exposed to the vicissitudes of the environment, if it has no vital purpose? How can we explain the evolutionary pressure that was brought to bear in preserving this situation when its disadvantages are apparently greater than any possible advantages?

Some have tried to solve this riddle by claiming that REM sleep becomes vital only in the critical stages of development of the central nervous system. This theory is linked to a psychiatrist named Howard Roffwarg, who was also a member of the first group of sleep researchers that formed around Dement and Rechtschaffen. According to Roffwarg and his colleagues, the fact that the actual amount of REM sleep is very great during the first few days after birth, and that this sleep probably also appears in the fetal stage, shows that it plays a vital role in the maturing stage of the nervous system. Studies conducted on animals showed that the normal development of the nervous system is conditional on the reception of sensory information at the critical stages of that development. Kittens that immediately after birth grew up in total darkness, with a complete absence of visual stimuli, showed signs of degeneration of nerve cells in the visual cerebral cortex. It is therefore probable that the role of REM sleep is to ensure that the cerebral cortex receives sensory stimuli, which are so necessary for the maturing of the nerve cells, during the critical development period. The brain stem, the development of which was completed before the maturing of the cerebral cortex, is responsible for bombarding it with sensory stimuli during REM sleep. As it is almost impossible to prevent REM sleep for long periods in animals immediately after birth, we cannot test what came to be called "the ontogenetic theory of REM sleep."

In my own attempts to provide an answer to the riddle of REM sleep, I shall avail myself of the thoughts of other researchers. When Nathaniel Kleitman was asked, "What is the role of sleep?" his rejoinder would be, "Tell me what the role of wakefulness is and then I shall explain the role of sleep." Can we find a role of any kind for the state of wakefulness? Does the question hold any physiological meaning beyond its philosophical significance? My own views on the role of REM sleep are similar to Kleitman's approach to the role of sleep in general. In my view, REM sleep was not created from the outset in order to satisfy a particular need. I believe that it is an unavoidable result of the transition from interrupted, or polyphasic, sleep, which characterizes most animals and the human infant during the first months of its life, to uninterrupted and continuous, or monophasic, sleep.

The eminent Harvard biologist Stephen Jay Gould published a fascinating essay called "Natural Selection and the Human Brain: Darwin vs. Wallace" in his book *The Panda's Thumb*. Gould placed himself firmly on Charles Darwin's side in the latter's great debate with Alfred Russel Wallace on the evolution of the human brain. This debate revolved around the question of whether the human brain could also be viewed as an evolutionary product according to the principles of natural selection, or whether, as Wallace claimed, the brain was created with the help of divine intervention. Gould claimed that natural selection could build an organ "for" a defined function or group of functions, but that this "purpose" did not necessarily determine the full potential of the organ. A structure designed for a specific purpose can perform, because of its complexity, many other tasks. He concludes his essay thus: "I do not deny that nature has its harmonies. But structure also has its latent capacities. Built for one thing, it can do others—and in this flexibility lies both the messiness and the hope for our lives."

When I read Gould's essay, I found it fitted my way of thinking about REM sleep perfectly. It reminded me of Kleitman's claim regarding the relationship between REM sleep and dreams. Kleitman claimed that dreams were only a by-product of the high level of arousal of the cerebral cortex during REM sleep, just as speech was a by-product of the air movements that agitate the vocal cords when breathing. Therefore, said Kleitman, it cannot be argued that REM sleep was created in order to allow people to dream. In my own estimation, REM sleep made its first appearance on the evolutionary stage as a solution to the problem of uniting the numerous and brief periods of sleep into a single continuous period. Only later were many other varied roles added that "exploited" its "latent capacities," to use Gould's words.

On what, then, do I base my claim that REM sleep is the "glue" that binds polyphasic sleep to the monophasic kind? First, as I mentioned earlier, the physiological characteristics of REM sleep bear a greater similarity to the characteristics of wakefulness than to those of sleep. Cerebral arousal is reflected in the brain waves, rapid eye movements, and a lack of stability in the autonomic nervous system that is reminiscent of emotional conditions when awake. During REM sleep, the brain loses control of the regulatory mechanisms. This phenomenon can be explained in the same way. Eliot Phillipson of the University of Toronto, who has made a significant contribution to the understanding of the function of the regulatory mechanisms of breathing during sleep, showed that respiratory control during REM sleep is performed by the same brain mechanism that is active during wakefulness, and not by the brain stem's "automatic" mechanisms which oversee breathing in the other sleep stages.

Second, the longest duration of a REM sleep occurs at the time when sleep becomes consolidated into monophasic sleep, during the first months of life. Its relative amount then gradually decreases. Moreover, unlike the adult's first REM sleep, which always appears after about an hour and a half of sleep of stages 1, 2, 3, and 4, the infant's REM sleep may appear immediately after it has fallen asleep. It was this phenomenon that caught Eugene Aserinsky's eye and led him directly to the discovery of REM sleep.

Several findings support the claim that REM sleep is a "gate" to wakefulness during sleep, a gate through which it is very easy to wake up, even without the help of an alarm clock. In 1975, two master's degree students, Jacob Zomer and Arieh Oksenberg, conducted an experiment in my laboratory. They tested the ability of a person to awaken at a predetermined time without the help of an alarm clock or any other external factor. Many people claim to be able to do this, so we devoted a great deal of time to finding reliable subjects. The findings of the study verified the subjects' claims. The precision of their awakenings was most impressive; most of them awakened some ten minutes before or after the target times. But no less impressive was the observation that the majority of these awakenings were from REM sleep. If, for example, we asked a subject to wake up at 3:30 A.M., he would awaken from the REM sleep closest to the target time—say, at 3:15 A.M. These findings were later substantiated by further studies conducted in the United States and Japan. We can conclude that in some way or other, we can maintain contact with reality during REM sleep and even decide when to wake up with the help of internal signals. Interestingly, in one of the earliest theories of REM sleep, Fred Snyder proposed that REM sleep has evolved to allow the organism periodic scanning of possible signs of danger in the environment.

Further proof that REM sleep is a gateway to wakefulness in the continuity of sleep was provided by observations in free-running subjects who were completely isolated from environmental time markers. Under these conditions, they awoke from REM sleep numerous times, far more than they awakened from it when they slept in their natural environment. Similar observations were reported by Tom Wehr of the National Institute of Mental Health, who investigated the sleep of subjects living in prolonged periods of darkness.

Spontaneous awakening from REM sleep as a response to a demand to wake up at a predetermined time, and spontaneous awakening from REM sleep under conditions of isolation from time markers, both show that REM sleep allows a smooth and rapid transition from sleep to wakefulness, which supports the claim that REM sleep can be viewed as a gate to wakefulness during sleep.

Further findings at the Technion Sleep Laboratory demonstrated an additional advantage in awakening from REM sleep. When we examined how people functioned after awakening from REM sleep, we found that they performed very well at tasks which included orientation in space. These tasks, which are controlled by the right hemisphere of the brain, were performed with a lesser success rate after awakening from the deep sleep of stages 3 and 4. In other words, a person awakening from REM sleep is immediately oriented in his surroundings, which is of cardinal importance to a smooth transition from sleep to wakefulness.

The existence of these "gates to wakefulness" in sleep, which manifests itself in the ability of a person to wake up easily and immediately be at the peak of sensory awareness, is similar to that of the "gates to sleep" during wakefulness, which we have already discussed. With sleep gates, like the secondary gate to sleep which appears during the afternoon, it is relatively easy to fall asleep. The existence of gates to wakefulness during sleep and gates to sleep during wakefulness provides greater flexibility in the transition from sleep to wakefulness, and vice versa. And although the gates are not always exploited for passage to and from sleep, they are used to make all the necessary physiological changes that ensure rapid and efficient awakening or falling asleep, whenever the need arises.

REM sleep is therefore not simply a caprice of the brain or a grandiose evolutionary mistake. In all likelihood it is one of the most awe-inspiring examples of the flexibility of evolution and its ability fully to exploit the latent characteristics of existing conditions and structures. Although REM sleep was not intended to play a part in the control and regulation of instincts, the consolidation of memory traces, the regulation of cerebral arousal, or the creation of dreams, its particular characteristics, as a gate to wakefulness while asleep, fulfill many and varied roles.

# Sleep Centers

Numerous assumptions have been aired throughout history regarding the location of the organ responsible for sleep—from Aristotle's theory that the cooling of the heart was the reason for sleep, to the belief of Plato and Galen that sleep was caused by the "blocking of the brain's pores by the foul vapors of food," to the theories of "too much blood" and "too little blood" which were propounded in the nineteenth century. The first suggestion that a special center in the brain caused sleep was made by Constantin von Economo, and it was related to a terrible epidemic at the beginning of the twentieth century. The story of encephalitis lethargica, or "sleeping sickness," has recently been revivified with the publication of *Awakenings* by the neurologist Oliver Sacks. Sacks's book tells the story in a most thrilling way, but it is a pity that he concentrated solely on the sufferers and did not cast any light on the multifaceted personality of von Economo, the discoverer of the disease which also bears his name, who could easily be the subject of a full-length movie.

Von Economo was born in Romania in 1876 to an aristocratic family of Macedonian extraction. Young Constantin was a gifted child who spoke several languages fluently, and although his father had sent him to Vienna to study engineering, he went against his father's wishes and turned to medicine instead. He graduated with honors in 1901 and went on to specialize in psychiatry in Paris and Munich. On completion of his studies, he returned to Vienna and began work at a psychiatric clinic, where he spent the rest of his life.

Von Economo was a pioneer in aviation as well as medicine. As there was not a single airplane in the whole of Austria in 1907, he began his aeronautical career in balloons. By 1908 he had achieved one of his life's dreams: he completed a pilot's course in France, was awarded his license, and brought the first airplane to be seen over Vienna back to Austria. Not surprisingly, von Economo became Austria's first military pilot and saw action in the First World War, his primary mission being observation flights over the Alps. His military flying career was cut short by the death of his brother in battle, after which he returned to Vienna as a doctor specializing in head injuries.

Von Economo discovered sleeping sickness in 1917, following the sudden outbreak of the mysterious disease the previous winter. In January of that year, von Economo saw the first patient who was suffering from a high temperature, hallucinations, impaired vision, and excessive sleepiness. This patient was quickly followed by another six. As the disease manifested itself in varying forms, these patients had been diagnosed as suffering from a variety of diseases, from schizophrenia to Parkinson's disease. It was here that von Economo's extraordinary clinical talents came to the fore. He immediately pinpointed the factor common to all the cases, and in May 1917 he published a scientific article on his newly discovered disease: sleeping sickness, or encephalitis lethargica. In the article, he wrote that the thread connecting the cases was the serious sleep disorders, which manifested themselves in the form of excessive sleepiness that lasted for weeks and months, or a total lack of sleep that ended in death.

The disease spread throughout the world and caused the deaths of more than five million people in the space of ten years. In 1927 it disappeared with the same mysterious suddenness with which it had arisen. The disease's effect on sleep was dramatic; approximately one-third of the patients fell asleep for extended periods, and it was impossible to awaken them. The majority died while still asleep. Some suffered from the opposite symptom—a total inability to fall asleep even with the help of drugs. A small number of patients sank into a sleep from which, something like Rip van Winkle, they awoke years later! Sacks found some of these patients in an institution for the chronically sick and treated them with L-dopa (levodopa), which awakened them from their endless sleep as though a magic wand had been waved over them. Unfortunately, the end of this story was not as happy as its beginning, and Sacks was forced to stop the L-dopa treatment because of the serious side-effects it produced.

Von Economo began an exhaustive study of the brains of patients who had died of sleeping sickness and found signs of brain damage in all of them. In the patients who had suffered disorders in their sleep, the damage was always located in the same area of the brain, very close to the hypothalamus. This brain center is, among other things, responsible for eating and drinking, as well as for the functioning of the autonomic nervous system. When the clinical symptoms included excessive sleepiness, the damage was located in the posterior part of the hypothalamus, and when the symptoms showed lack of sleep, the damage was in the anterior area. Von Economo concluded that the area adjacent to the hypothalamus was linked to the control of sleep. He assumed that the "sleep center" was actively responsible for the neural, physical, and behavioral changes that occurred during the transition from wakefulness to sleep. He rejected the possibility that the activation of the center was related to the blocking of the sensory information channels, but hypothesized that the compounds produced during wakefulness, which Henri Pieron had named "hypnotoxins" at the beginning of the century, were those that activated the sleep center.

Von Economo postulated that the principal objective of the sleep center was to prevent the "toxification" of the entire brain by the hypnotoxins. This, according to him, was the principal function of sleep itself. Once the disposal process of the hypnotoxins had been completed, sleep came to an end. Von Economo also recognized the effects of habits and learning processes upon sleep and its control. The reasons for this were that sleep often appeared without any feelings of tiredness and that it was a simple matter to stop sleep in the middle, before the conclusion of hypnotoxin removal process. It would become clear many years later that Siamese twins who share a common circulatory system are not always asleep and awake at the same time. This observation is incompatible with the claim that the main cause of sleep is the compounds which are carried in the bloodstream and which activate the sleep center.

Sadly, von Economo did not live to see his theories on brain centers that control sleep substantiated in controlled studies. In 1931, he died in his sleep of a heart attack at age fifty-five.

## THE ISOLATED BRAIN

Von Economo's observations and theories on the location of the sleep center had a great effect on his contemporary brain researchers. Numerous researchers dissected the areas which he had described as being of great significance to sleep. They tried to induce sleeping sickness artificially but were unsuccessful. And yet the discovery of brain waves by Hans Berger, and their widespread use as a research tool by the end of the thirties, brought about a dramatic change in the research techniques used to investigate the function of the brain. Researchers no longer needed to depend solely on the appearance and behavior of the laboratory animal; they could now determine objectively whether it was awake or asleep. However, the interpretation of the findings was not always accurate. Frederic Bremer, a Belgian researcher who followed von Economo's observations closely, was the first to conduct experiments on the separation of the cerebrum from the brain stem. To his amazement, immediately after the effects of the anesthesia had dissipated, the animal showed all the signs of sleep, including the characteristic brain waves of sleep. This was diametrically opposed to the results of separating the brain from the spinal column—in other words, a situation in which the brain and the brain stem remained joined but were separated from the rest of the body. This would cause uninterrupted wakefulness without sleep. Years later, Bremer admitted that had he been anatomy-oriented, he might have reached the conclusion that the brain stem, between the spinal cord and the cerebrum, housed a mechanism that was vital for maintaining the alertness of the cerebrum. This was the mechanism that was separated from the cerebrum as a result of the surgery. And yet Bremer was a prisoner of the idea that sleep was a passive condition caused by the isolation of the brain from the sensory information channels. He interpreted the signs of sleep thus: the isolation of the brain from the brain stem caused sleep because of the separation of the nerve channels which carried sensation from the sensory organs. More than ten years passed before the existence of a special mechanism which controlled the level of alertness of the cerebrum in the brain stem was proved. This mechanism has no need at all of sensory information in order to maintain the condition of wakefulness.

Although von Economo did not witness the great strides made in brain research from the middle of the twentieth century, his writings show that he was fully aware of the earlier experiments conducted by the Swiss scientist Walter Rudolf Hess. Hess, who was almost the same age as von Economo, completed his medical studies in 1905 and went on to specialize in ophthalmology. He quickly came to abhor the monotony of his new profession and accepted a research post at a Zurich physiological institute. His studies focused on the way in which the brain controlled autonomous physiological systems like blood pressure and the function of the digestive system. In order to study how the brain controlled the various systems, he developed an innovative research technique: by inserting extremely delicate electrodes into the brain of an animal, he was able to stimulate the brain electrically. As these experiments were conducted on animals that were awake and able to wander freely around their cages, Hess was able to document very precisely how the electrical stimuli affected their behavior.

Unlike von Economo, who discovered encephalitis lethargica after observing only seven patients, Hess continued his experiments for no less than twenty-five years. With the publication of his conclusions in 1949, he was awarded the Nobel Prize for medicine for his achievements in understanding the principles of cerebral control of the various physiological systems. In one of his articles, Hess admitted that he had not really intended to study sleep but had begun to do so almost against his will after a number of cases had shown that electrical stimuli had caused the laboratory animal to fall asleep. That both he and his mother suffered from insomnia probably contributed to his interest in sleep. In his paper "Biological Order and Brain Organization," he described one of his experiments thus: "Experiment 180 (15 March 1935): Friendly animal. Insertion of the electrodes causes no symptoms. Stimulus with 1 volt for 30 seconds also has no effect. In contrast, increasing the intensity of the stimulus to 2 volts for 30–45 seconds has clear-cut effect. After two or three repetitions the cat assumes the typical position of sleep and falls asleep. This occurs even while stimulation is in progress. Her pupils are maximally narrowed and her behavior corresponds in every respect to that of a sleeping animal."

The electrodes which had caused the cat to fall asleep were inserted into the area of the brain identified by von Economo as the possible location of the sleep center, in the anterior part of the hypothalamus.

Little has changed since then. Hess devoted the last part of his life to an uncompromising and ultimately victorious struggle on behalf of the antivivisection movement in Switzerland.

## FATAL INSOMNIA: THE ROLE OF THE THALAMUS

In recent years there has been a growing recognition of yet another brain structure that plays an important role in sleep. The egg-shaped thalamus at the core of the brain is the main station linking the input arriving from the sense organs to the sensory areas in the cortex. Although Hess first called attention to the possible role of the thalamus in sleep, the excitement over the discoveries of the executive mechanisms of REM and non-REM sleep in the brain stem (to be described shortly) have left the thalamus relatively unexplored.

It was the clinical acumen of Elio Lugaresi, from Bologna, which pushed the thalamus onto center stage as a sleep-related brain structure. A fifty-three-year-old industrial manager consulted Lugaresi and his colleagues, complaining of increasing difficulty in falling asleep. The insomnia was associated with other symptoms such as constipation, increasing activity of the autonomic nervous system in the form of sweating, and higher heart rate, blood pressure, and body temperature. Some months after the initial appearance of these symptoms, insomnia had become almost total, and the manager's waking hours were interspersed with vivid dreamlike episodes. Gradually the patient lost contact with the people around him, and he died nine months after the onset of his symptoms. His father and two sisters died in the same manner.

In these cases, too, the inability to sleep culminating in total insomnia was dramatic, justifying the name given to the disease—fatal familial insomnia. Strikingly, in all four cases postmortem brain examination revealed severe degeneration of the anterior part of the thalamus. Since in two of the patients the lesions were almost exclusively limited to the thalamus, Lugaresi and his colleagues concluded that the anterior part of the thalamus plays a major role in sleep regulation. Later studies have shown that fatal familial insomnia is an inherited disease and is always fatal. Lugaresi's clinical observations agreed with experimental evidence.

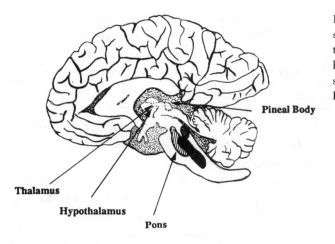

Fig. 28. The brain
stem areas that con-
trol wakefulness (in
black), non-REM
sleep (striated), and
REM sleep (dotted)

It is well documented that spindle brain waves, which are the electro-
encephalographic landmark for sleep onset, originate in the thalamus.


## THE WAKEFULNESS CENTER

Very much like the discovery of REM sleep, the discovery of a wakefulness center in the brain was pure chance. Giuseppe Moruzzi, a neurophysiologist from Pisa, and his colleague, Horace Magoun of Chicago,
had never intended to study the brain center that controls wakefulness.
Their objective apparently had been to study the neural paths which lead
from the cerebellum to the motor cerebral cortex. They therefore inserted
electrodes into the brain stem area which they viewed as a relay station
along the neural paths that connected the two areas. When they activated
the electrical stimulus, they observed, probably to their surprise, that the
stimulus had caused brain waves that indicated tense alertness. As the
stimulus electrodes were not located close to the sensory paths which
conduct information to the brain, they assumed that they had stimulated
an unknown neural path which had activated the entire cerebral cortex
and not merely a small, specific part of it. There can be no doubt that
the experiment had been observed by the right people! They immediately
assessed the significance of their discovery. Magoun, who had previously

studied the brain mechanisms related to sleep, knew that wide areas of the brain stem, which were still very much terra incognita for neurophysiologists, were related to the control of the autonomous nervous system. Moruzzi, who had studied neurophysiology under Frederic Bremer, was fully conversant with the recording of brain waves and their significance in the determination of states of sleep and wakefulness.

Moruzzi and Magoun summed up their discovery in the following way: "Stimulation of the reticular formation [the name they gave to the stimulated area] of the cerebral cortex causes variations in the brain waves. The high, slow waves disappear and are replaced by rapid, low ones. These waves are not the result of stimulating the sensory paths that traverse the cerebral cortex. The arousal response to stimulation of the reticular formation and the arousal response to natural stimulation (such as noise or touch) were the same. It is worthy of note that continuous activity in the brain stem reticular formation can explain the condition of wakefulness. A decrease in its activity, either natural or through drugs, illness or surgery, can cause sleep, somnolence or pathological sleep."

When they studied the structure of the reticular formation, they saw that it was an integrative system that receives information from all the paths that lead sensation to the brain and from all the motor paths that take orders from the brain to the muscles. In this way, the formation can delay or expedite the passage of all kinds of information.

How, then, does the transition from wakefulness to sleep occur? What is the mechanism that activates and retards the reticular formation? At least two separate mechanisms are capable of retarding the wakefulness mechanism, the first of which I have already discussed in my description of the sleep centers in the hypothalamus area. These mechanisms are connected by neural paths to the reticular formation, and through them the sleep center can retard the activity of the arousal center and cause falling asleep.

There is another center located in the area which joins the spinal column to the brain stem. This center was discovered in 1949 at Moruzzi's laboratory by Yochanan Magnes, a young student who later became a professor at the Hebrew University of Jerusalem. This mechanism is located in the lower portion of the brain stem, in an area called the rhombencephalon. Electrical stimulation of the area put a laboratory animal to sleep immediately, while its destruction caused continued lack of sleep. Whichever mechanism signals the onset of sleep, it must activate the thalamic sleep structure which starts producing spindles marking the onset of sleep.

## REM SLEEP MECHANISMS

I have so far described the brain mechanisms which are linked to the falling-asleep process and maintenance of the level of wakefulness. The discoveries that revealed how the mechanisms which control REM sleep and that of other stages worked were also made, in the main, by chance. At the beginning of his career in research, Michel Jouvet furthered his studies with Magoun at the Brain Research Institute in Los Angeles. On his return to the University of Lyons, his principal field of interest was the location of the brain mechanisms related to simple learning processes. In order to study the learning mechanisms without any possible influences, he conducted his experiments on cats whose brains had been separated from the brain stem by a technique similar to that used by Bremer. To his great surprise, he found that the animals' muscle tonus disappeared completely every thirty to forty minutes for a period of five to six minutes, without any form of outside intervention. During these periods of "paralysis," high and sharp waves appeared in the pons area of the brain stem, together with agitated movements of the cats' whiskers.

Numerous researchers, including Bremer himself, who conducted similar studies presumably witnessed the same phenomenon, because experiments in which the brain was isolated from the brain stem were very common in the first half of the twentieth century. But not all researchers possessed either Jouvet's curiosity or his spark of genius. Once he had observed the periods of paralysis, he immediately assumed that they were identical to the periods of REM sleep which had already been described in humans by Aserinsky and Kleitman, and later in cats by Dement. Two experiments proved him right. In cats whose brains were normal, the period of paralysis and the bursts of high, sharp waves were also accompanied by brain wave activity characteristic of REM sleep, rapid eye movements, and twitching of the limbs and whiskers. These phenomena were completely identical to Dement's earlier observations in cats. In the second experiment he found that it was possible to prevent the period of paralysis and its accompanying changes by precise surgery on the lateral section of the brain stem. However, this surgery did not impair the sleep characterized by slow, high brain waves. This was how Jouvet discovered that the mechanism that controls paradoxical sleep in cats was located in the brain stem in the pons area.

The case of Y. H., which I discussed above, proved beyond doubt that the location of the mechanism responsible for REM sleep in humans was identical to its location in cats. The shell splinter that had lodged in Y. H.'s brain stem was in exactly the same location that Jouvet had indicated in his operations as the site of the control mechanism of paradoxical sleep in cats. Jouvet later used techniques for the chemical mapping of the brain, which had first been discovered at about that time, to show that the area connected with the control of REM sleep was rich in noradrenalin and acetylcholine neurotransmitters (chemical compounds which are secreted by the nerve ends that carry nerve impulses). The adjacent areas, called raphe nuclei, are, according to Jouvet's experiments, related to sleep characterized by slow, high-voltage waves and are rich in the neurotransmitter serotonin.

# Sleep Medicine
## *The First Steps*

After I completed my doctorate in physiological psychology at the University of Florida, I moved west to the University of California in San Diego for postdoctoral studies at the Department of Psychiatry Sleep Laboratory. The laboratory head was Dan Kripke, a psychiatrist who had "majored" in computers as a hobby years before we all became experts in that particular field. At the time, Kripke was interested in biological rhythms, a subject also close to my heart. He managed to obtain a research grant for me from a pharmaceutical company so that I could continue my studies in his laboratory. Although I had undertaken a study on drug therapy for insomnia, I still had a great many free nights in which I was able to study other subjects and gain clinical experience at the same time.

At the beginning of the seventies, relatively few people had laboratory experience in the diagnosis of sleep disorders. The few American sleep laboratories that undertook clinical examination were chiefly engaged in testing the effects of sleeping drugs. In fact, the pharmaceutical companies were the first to discover the hidden potential of laboratory sleep recordings. Instead of relying on the patient's subjective report on the efficacy of the drug, it became possible to obtain an authenticated opinion based on objective observations and evaluations from "sleep specialists." It goes without saying that the mere fact that the various drugs were tested in a laboratory was of great promotional value. As the San Diego sleep laboratory was located in a hospital, I was able to meet a great many people that year who suffered from insomnia, and also a few patients who suffered from narcolepsy, a sleep disorder which manifests itself in involuntary falling asleep and muscle paralysis during the day. After I had seen the first few patients, it became clear that the question What is a good sleep? is not easy to answer.

Most people do not pay a great deal of attention to their sleep unless they suddenly discover that something is wrong with it. The "something wrong" can happen to them or even to others who are close to them. The disruption may occur in a number of ways: sleep can be a long time in coming, be interrupted many times during the night, or even be terminated in the middle of the night. Sleep can also be very demanding and force itself upon us when we don't want it.

Determining the type and cause of sleep disorders starts with interviewing patients. When asked how they have slept, they reply according to their feelings and what the coming day has in store for them. They do not "analyze" the structure of their sleep, the number of REM periods, or the duration of deep sleep. We feel that we have slept well if we wake up feeling refreshed and clear-headed, and if we see the world around us in all its clear and sharply focused colors. After awakening from a sleep like that, our customary "good morning" takes on a special meaning.

There are, however, people to whom such feelings are almost completely unknown. They experience them, but only rarely. Some struggle nightly with their sleep. They spend long hours in bed attempting to fall asleep, or fall asleep rapidly only to wake up after an hour or so wide awake, unable to return to sleep. Others, although they fall asleep without difficulty and think they have slept the entire night, nevertheless awaken with completely different feelings: their heads are heavy, their bodies fatigued, their thinking slow, and their senses dull. "Sleeping tires me out," they claim, and "The longer I sleep, the more tired I wake up." These people require quite a few minutes in order to "recover" from sleep.

Apart from nonrefreshing and insufficient sleep, other things can go wrong at night. Some people display behavior that should have no place in sleep, such as sleepwalking and talking or grinding the teeth. These are all examples of automatic behavior that occurs during sleep without the sleeper's awareness.

What separates the sleep of those who wake up with a smile on their faces and that of those who wake up tired—the "good" sleepers from the "bad" sleepers? As I shall show, there are many and varied reasons, mental and physical, for this difference.

## "DOCTOR, I HAVEN'T SLEPT A WINK ALL NIGHT": INSOMNIA

> What is our insomnia but the mad obstinacy of our mind in
> manufacturing thoughts and trains of reasoning, syllogisms
> and definitions of its own, refusing to abdicate in favor of that
> divine stupidity of closed eyes, or the wise folly of dreams?
> The man who cannot sleep . . . refuses more or less
> consciously to entrust himself to the flow of things.
> —Marguerite Yourcenar, *Memoirs of Hadrian,*
> trans. Grace Frick

We have seen in previous chapters that there is a great variation in the amount of sleep different people need. For some, five to six hours are sufficient, while others sleep nine hours or more. The immense range of sleep hours in a normal population makes a clear definition of insomnia extremely difficult. Does the person who sleeps six hours every night but is convinced that he should be getting eight hours of sleep suffer from insomnia just like the person who sleeps eight hours but is dissatisfied with less than ten? In our clinical work at the Technion Sleep Laboratory, I have met both categories of people, and all were convinced that they were suffering from a severe sleep disorder. Diagnosing insomnia is therefore mainly based upon the patients' subjective feelings regarding the amount and quality of their sleep, but the diagnosis is of course aided by objective laboratory recordings. People assess the quality of their sleep according to their views about sleep and its importance. Sometimes, much to the chagrin of the sleep researcher, there is absolutely no correlation at all between the subject's feelings and beliefs and the sleep laboratory's findings.

In diagnosing the causes of insomnia, particular attention should be paid to four points:

First, what does the insomnia sufferer really mean when he says, "Doctor, I haven't slept a wink all night"? This complaint can cover a multitude of vastly different sleep disorders. There are many forms of insomnia, the most common of which are difficulty in falling asleep, frequent awakening, and a combination of both. Some other forms, including waking up in the early hours of the morning and awakening at regular intervals throughout the night, are less common. It is of cardinal importance to clarify the specific characteristic of the sleep disorder because this information can have some bearing on the reason behind the disorder itself. This clarification is the first step in deciding upon suitable treatment.

Second, the onset of the disorder must be established, for the time at which the disorder began is also of great importance to the diagnosis. There will be a vast difference between the diagnosis of a patient's disorder which has only recently begun—resulting, say, from an important event in his life, such as a death in the family, being made redundant, or a divorce—and that of a patient whose disorder began many years ago and which is linked, for example, to a chronic disease or even to his childhood.

Third, we must try to establish the severity of the disorder. This varies from person to person, and the variations are often extreme. In some cases the disorder manifests itself night after night, while in others it appears and disappears. If the disorder does indeed tend to come and go, the conditions under which it does so must be clarified: Are they linked to vacations, long journeys, or possibly other stressful life events?

Finally, the degree to which the sleep disorder affects behavior and functioning during the day is also of great importance. The approach to the sleep disorder will be completely different if the patient complains that he is totally incapable of functioning during the day because he "can't sleep at night," or if he views the disorder simply as something bothersome that does not affect his functional level during the day.

These four characteristics—the form the disorder takes, the circumstances and time of its appearance, the degree of severity, and its effect on daily functioning—aid us in making our initial diagnosis of the source of the disorder and deciding on suitable treatment. Indeed, when someone comes to the Technion Sleep Laboratory complaining of insomnia, we place great emphasis on the initial interview. In many cases, we are able to forgo a night examination in the laboratory and make a diagnosis on the basis of the interview alone.

I shall now describe the main diagnoses of insomnia disorders and the characteristics of each one.

## SITUATIONAL INSOMNIA

Sleep is an accurate barometer of the subject's mental condition, respond-ing rapidly to situations of tension and anxiety, sometimes even before any other bodily system does so.

When sleep disorders begin as the result of a significant event in the life of the subject, such as a family or a financial crisis, the insomniac will be able to pinpoint the date of the first appearance of the disorder. For example: "Since March 1, 1991, when I started divorce proceedings against my husband, I can't manage to fall asleep at night," or "Since my wife died I can't sleep more than two or three hours a night." I should say at the outset that there is nothing out of the ordinary in the appearance of sleep disorders as a reaction to significant events in our lives. By their very nature they cause overarousal and fretful thoughts which disturb our peace of mind, especially when we are not occupied. "What is our in-somnia but the mad obstinacy of our mind in manufacturing thoughts and trains of reasoning, syllogisms and definitions of its own . . . ?" to repeat Hadrian's definition of insomnia in Marguerite Yourcenar's book. The high level of arousal and the worrisome thoughts, too, interfere with the normal process of falling asleep and thus prevent sleep. Therefore, in most cases of situational insomnia patients complain more of difficulty in falling asleep and less of waking up while asleep. Once they have finally fallen asleep, they usually sleep well until the morning. Situational insomnia, the causes of which are known and which began relatively recently, should therefore be regarded as part of the totality of mental reactions to a stressful situation and to anxiety.

## SLEEP UNDER THE THREAT OF MISSILE ATTACK

In most cases situational insomnia affects people who are faced with personal difficulties. There are unusual situations, however, when large groups of people are bound in the same stressful situation and may be condemned together to sleepless nights. One of the most striking exam-ples of situational insomnia which I have witnessed occurred during the Gulf War. Thirty-eight of the thirty-nine Scud missile attacks on Israel took place during the evening and at night. Even to the Israelis, who are no strangers to war, the Scud threat was something out of the ordinary:

the warning time before an imminent attack was short, and the fear that the missiles might be carrying chemical warheads was very real. Because of the possibility of a chemical attack, unprecedented civil defense procedures were put into force, procedures which by their very nature carried the threat of extreme danger. It was therefore hardly surprising that many people were frightened of going to sleep. Their main fears were either that the siren sounding the alert would not wake them up, or that their awakening would be slow and confused, thereby preventing them from taking the necessary precautions: putting on a gas mask and closing themselves up in a sealed room. Undoubtedly the general anxiety caused by the war also had its impact.

A survey conducted during this period showed that one-third of the adult population complained of difficulty in falling asleep and of frequent awakenings. These complaints were most common in the Haifa and Tel Aviv areas, which were the main targets of the Scud attacks, and their frequency was three times higher than that of sleep-linked complaints recorded before the war. As the Sleep Laboratory was quite naturally closed down during the war, we used the time for objective study of the effects of the missile attacks on the sleep of Israel's population. Using mobile equipment which enabled us to record the sleep of subjects in their own homes, we observed twenty adults and fifty children for the duration of the war. The results were surprising: On comparing sleep recordings made on nights when attacks took place with those made on uneventful nights, we found that, apart from awakening during the attacks themselves, adults and children alike experienced no real disturbance to sleep! Our initial doubts regarding the sensitivity of the home recorders were dispelled when we checked what had occurred to subjects who had slept in the Sleep Laboratory.

Once it had became clear that the war would not be over within a few days, we decided to renew our sleep tests after one of the rooms had been fitted out as a sealed room to be used in the event of an attack. Ten subjects were tested in the Technion Sleep Laboratory during nights in which Israel was under missile attack. On those nights, when the alarm was sounded, the technicians woke the subjects, disconnected them from the recording equipment, helped them into their gas masks, and led them to the sealed room. I know of no other experiment in which sleep laboratory tests have been made on the effects of a night missile attack on

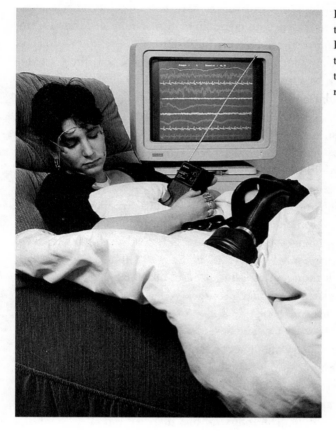

Fig. 29. Sleeping in
the Technion Sleep
Laboratory during
the Gulf War, with
the gas mask
nearby

the quality of sleep, and I doubt whether such an experiment will ever
be conducted again in the future. Those ten subjects will go down in the
history of science as the most courageous test group in the annals of sleep
research. The test results corresponded with our earlier findings: the
subjects' sleep, both before and after the attacks, did not differ at all
from the sleep of thousands of subjects who had slept in the laboratory
prior to the war. Once an attack was over and the all clear was sounded,
when the technicians took the subjects back to their rooms and recon-
nected them to the recording instruments, the longest sleep latency period
was twelve minutes!

How, then, can we reconcile the findings of the survey, which showed
a sharp rise in the incidence of insomnia, with the fact that objective

tests in both the laboratory and subjects' homes revealed no real sleep disorders? In my judgment, the complaints of insomnia generated a tremendous amount of media interest, which in turn fueled the feelings of anxiety. People were simply afraid of going to sleep, and their anxiety and apprehension was translated into complaints of difficulty in falling asleep and frequent awakenings from sleep. Yet from the moment they fell asleep, they slept uninterruptedly. Thus, once initiated, the sleep process was immune to waking feelings of anxiety and stress. To reduce people's fears, we had to reinforce their sense of security and reassure them that they would indeed wake up in the event of an attack, even in locations where the warning siren was completely inaudible.

During the third week of the war, a psychiatrist friend, Ehud Klein, called me asking for my help in a matter he regarded as urgent. He told me that he had contacted the chief engineer of Israel Radio and suggested that they leave one channel open every night as a "silent channel" which would start broadcasting only in the event of an attack. For reasons unknown to him, his suggestion had been received with no great enthusiasm, and he hoped that my prestige as a sleep researcher would help. I immediately called the chief engineer and tried to persuade him that implementing Klein's idea would encourage Israel's population to stand firm in the face of the attacks. The engineer's reply was vague, but the idea had already taken wing through the corridors of the Broadcasting Authority, and that same day I was asked to appear on the daily television program *A New Evening*. The interview had the required effect, and that very evening the "silent channel" went into operation. Surveys conducted during the war showed that more than half of Israel's population went to bed every night with the radio silently "broadcasting" by their bedsides. Many people testified that the "silent channel" had made a real difference to their sleep. They could now go to sleep safe in the knowledge that they would be awakened in good time in the event of a surprise night attack.

Situational insomnia does pass, however, once a change occurs in the external conditions that caused it, which is why it is also called temporary insomnia. Indeed, the impression made by the missile attacks disappeared with the cessation of hostilities. Today, the majority of Israelis have only dim memories of the Gulf War, which left few psychological marks or scars. I still wonder whether the silent-channel technique could be used to treat those sufferers from "fear of sleep" who are unable to detach themselves from the pressures of daily events.

Sufferers from situational insomnia need to be calmed and reassured; they should be told that their reaction is perfectly natural and does not indicate a mental disorder of any kind. There is a wide range of treatments for more severe cases where the sleep disorder prevents normal functioning during the day, but I shall expand on them later.

In surveys conducted on the incidence of sleep disorders in the general population, those who give an affirmative answer to the question Do you sometimes suffer from sleep disorders? are almost certainly referring to situational insomnia, especially when they reply "sometimes" or "frequently." According to surveys conducted in a wide range of countries, some 15–18 percent of the adult population suffer from insomnia at least "sometimes." Interestingly, in all the surveys women complain of insomnia more than men, and although there are many explanations for this disparity between the sexes regarding sleep complaints, I am not convinced that we are sure of its source. It is probable that the vulnerability of women's sleep reflects deep differences in personality structure and ways of reacting to stress. On the other hand, these differences may reflect sociological factors. At least in the past, men were considered to be "strong" as the bread winners and could not afford to be sick. If this sociological explanation is correct then the male/female difference should gradually diminish as the traditional sex roles change.

## CHRONIC INSOMNIA

Although insomnia can be a natural reaction to a stressful situation and does not necessarily indicate mental disorder, there is still a danger that it will become long-lasting and persistent, sometimes even after the crisis that caused it has long passed. This is chronic, not situational, insomnia. The circumstances under which situational insomnia becomes chronic vary from person to person. There are those who, after a few nights of insomnia caused by some crisis or other, "learn" not to sleep. This should come as no surprise, because the process of falling asleep itself also has many elements of "learned behavior" and conditioning. In an imaginative experiment, Barry Sterman and his colleagues at the University of California in Los Angeles have demonstrated that an electrical stimulus applied to the anterior area of a cat's hypothalamus—which, it will be remembered, von Economo identified as a sleep center—caused almost immediate sleep. The researchers sounded a note a few seconds before the electrical stimulus was applied to the sleep center. After thirty-eight times in which the note was coupled with the electrical stimulus, the cat's brain waves showed clear signs of sleep immediately after the note had been sounded and before the electrical stimulus was applied. After a further training period, the cat quickly fell asleep as soon as it heard the note.

This experiment proved that a neutral stimulus which previously had no effect on sleep exerted a radical influence on sleep after being coupled many times with an electrical stimulus that caused the test animal to fall asleep. In a similar way, a totality of stimuli activates the sleep mechanisms in humans who have no sleep problems; from brushing the teeth and various other presleep rituals to laying the head on the pillow. As I mentioned earlier, falling asleep in front of the television can be explained in much the same way. There are many people who start yawning almost reflexively the moment they sit in their television chair, irrespective of how tired they are.

With insomnia, however, the conditioning is reversed. Associations are created which link the totality of bedroom stimuli with different signs of anxiety, and these prevent and delay sleep. After insomniacs have gone to bed, fretful and restless, any stimulus that is associatively linked to sleep causes further restlessness. In marked contrast with Sterman's cats, which were conditioned to fall asleep the moment the note was sounded, the heart rate and blood pressure of these people increase when they simply think about sleeping at night. As they brush their teeth and put on their pajamas, their level of arousal has almost reached its zenith, and when they get into bed and cover themselves up, they experience the greatest anxiety of all. People who "learn" not to sleep become part of a vicious circle, for as their insomnia increases in severity, the conditioning becomes more stable and consequently more difficult to treat. The disorder may disappear once the sufferers sleep far away from their own homes and beds and do not encounter, prior to going to bed, the nightly stimuli which cause their anxieties. They are then able to fall asleep with no difficulty, even when they are connected to sleep laboratory recording equipment. This reinforces the notion that these people suffer from insomnia which is a result of conditioning.

People who take behavioral habits like telephone calls, preparation of tomorrow's schedule, or eating, which are not conducive to the process of falling asleep, to bed with them, are liable to suffer from insomnia in a similar conditioning process.

Not only the conditioning process is liable to turn situational insomnia into chronic insomnia. The structure of the subject's personality is another contributory factor in the embedding of insomnia.

Some people find it "difficult" to give up their sleep disorder, for it "serves" them in their relationships with other people in their environment. To them, sleep and all that it entails become the axis upon which their entire world revolves. They unwittingly invest all their thoughts and effort in it. Using their insomnia as a lever, they bend everyone around them to their will. The whole family is in a state of permanent anxiety: Will Mom or Dad be able to sleep tonight? How did they sleep last night? Is the new treatment helping? By using these tactics, people suffering from a sleep disorder are always the center of attention. It goes without saying that their status would change if the insomnia disappeared, and so it is difficult for them to give it up.

I found a rare and beautiful description of the use to which sleep disorders can be put in *Remembrance of Things Past.* Marcel Proust is describing his aunt: " 'I must not forget that I never slept a wink.' Never sleeping a wink was her great claim to distinction, and one admitted and respected in our household vocabulary: in the morning Françoise would not 'call' her, but would simply 'go in' to her; during the day, when my aunt wished to take a nap, we used to say just that she wished to 'be quiet' or to 'rest'; and in conversation she so far forgot herself as to say 'What woke me up?' or 'I dreamed that,' she would blush and at once correct herself" (from *Swann's Way,* trans. C. K. Scott Moncrieff and Terence Kilmartin).

The sometimes compulsive need to exploit sleep disorders is linked to the fact that the sufferer from chronic insomnia is usually guilty of wild exaggeration regarding the severity of his disorder. This is shown in its most extreme form in the sleep laboratory. When insomniacs are tested in the laboratory, they are asked, after waking up in the morning, to try to assess how they have slept, how many times they have woken up, and how much time elapsed until they fell asleep. Finding a chronic insomnia sufferer who does not err in his or her assessment of the severity of the sleep disorder is a rare occurrence indeed. The margin of error is frequently huge. I can recall cases in which people fell asleep moments after the lights in the laboratory were turned off, and yet in the morning estimated that it had taken them hours to fall asleep. Others spent the greater part of the night in a deep sleep and yet in the morning swore that they hadn't closed their eyes all night.

Some people, however, do indeed have a real problem distinguishing between sleep and wakefulness. In a study we conducted in the Sleep Laboratory on the reasons for sleep assessment errors, we found that in a number of cases the error was caused by waking up for brief periods of no more than a few minutes, which were perceived as prolonged periods of wakefulness. Thus, for example, a person who awoke at 2 A.M. for five minutes, and an hour later woke up for a further five minutes, joined both short periods of wakefulness into a prolonged period which seemed to have lasted at least an hour. Some improvement was observed in the sleep of a large number of cases once the subjects had been provided with accurate information on the quality of their sleep and the gross error in their assessments, and its origin, had been explained to them.

Another way in which situational insomnia is liable to turn into chronic insomnia is linked to the uncontrolled use of sleeping pills. As I shall show in detail in Chapter 15, most sleeping drugs have a limited effect. When a person feels a deterioration in his sleep, he goes to his doctor and asks for help. If the doctor is unaware of the limitations in the effectiveness of the sleeping pills, he may decide to increase the dosage, or the patient sometimes decides to increase it without consulting the doctor. But after two to three weeks, even drugs prescribed at a high dosage will cease to have any effect on the patient. Thus the vicious circle of sleeping pill use is drawn: "drug tolerance," deterioration in the quality of sleep, increased dosage, again the appearance of tolerance and a further increase in dosage, and so on. After a few months, despite the increased dosage of drugs, the insomnia becomes chronic. Any attempt to stop medication produces withdrawal symptoms, including severe sleep disorders, nightmares, and great anxiety during the day. Those who are unable to face withdrawal return to sleeping pills, this time with an even higher dosage, or prepare "cocktails" of several types of drugs. This series of events was characteristic of many insomniacs tested in the laboratory, some of whom consumed drug cocktails every night. I recall two people who, before my very eyes, swallowed a mixture of eight different types of drugs before their sleep test in the laboratory! Both had a history of more than thirty years of severe insomnia.

Not all insomniacs are the victims of anxiety, stress, or maladaptive habits in the bedroom. A few report that they have suffered from a life-long inability to fall asleep. This form of insomnia is called "idiopathic" or "primary insomnia." Using the term *idiopathic* is an acknowledgment that we do not know much about the origin or causes of this form of insomnia.

Primary insomnia can be tormenting. Axel Munthe, the celebrated physician and author of *The Story of San Michele,* suffered from life-long insomnia. Even his great talent of hypnotizing patients, which he learned from Jean-Martin Charcot at La Salpêtrière in Paris, did not help him conquer his own insomnia: "Soon I ceased to sleep altogether, an attack of insomnia set in, so terrible that it nearly made me go off my head. Insomnia does not kill its man unless he kills himself—sleeplessness is the most common cause of suicide. But it kills his joie de vivre, it saps his strength, it sucks the blood from his brain and from his heart as a vampire. It makes him remember during the night what he was meant to forget in blissful sleep. It makes him forget during the day what he meant to remember. . . . Voltaire was right when he placed sleep in the same level as hope."

Most probably, people with this form of insomnia suffer from some abnormalities in the brain control mechanisms of sleep and wakefulness. These may be related to overactivation of the waking mechanism that interferes with the transition from wakefulness to sleep, or to a deficient activity of the sleep mechanism. In our experience, most of these patients respond poorly to sleep medications, as well as to other forms of treatment. Yet most, like Munthe, come to terms with their poor sleep. I vividly remember a fifty-year-old father and his twenty-year-old son who told me that they met regularly at 4 A.M. in the kitchen because of life-long insomnia. In both of them the insomnia began at a very young age and resisted any form of treatment.

# Treating Insomnia

"Hold him there, and take him away, for I'll make him sleep there tonight out of the air."

"By God," said the lad, "your worship can no more make me sleep in prison than make me king!"

"Well, why can't I make you sleep in prison?" asked Sancho.

"Now, my Lord Governor," answered the youth, "suppose your worship orders me to be taken to prison, and has me loaded with fetters and chains there and put in a cell, laying the jailer under heavy penalties to carry out your orders, and not let me out; all the same if I don't wish to sleep, and stay awake all night without closing an eyelid, will your worship with all your power be able to make me sleep if I don't choose to?"

—Cervantes, *The Adventures of Don Quixote*, trans.
J. M. Cohen

The dialogue between Don Quixote's squire, Sancho Panza, who had been appointed governor of Barataria by the duke, and the young boy who had been arrested on a charge of vagrancy and who turns out to be both witty and wise, sums up the central problem of the treatment of insomnia. It is impossible to force people to sleep against their will. Sleep must come to us by itself. Like surfers who carefully maneuver themselves into position to wait for a high wave, we can only prepare ourselves better in order to allow sleep to appear. Difficulty in falling asleep indicates that something is wrong with the sleep preparation process. The objective of all the treatments is therefore removing the obstacles and helping patients get ready for sleep so that the transition between wakefulness and sleep will be smooth. When the arousal level is high, and this manifests itself in tense muscles, "palpitations," and uncontrollable and worrisome thoughts, the falling-asleep process is impeded. Therefore, any technique that decreases arousal is likely to be of help in treating insomnia. These techniques include medication, relaxation, biofeedback, autohypnosis, and even the taking of measures to improve sleep hygiene. I shall begin with the non-medicinal techniques.

There are numerous relaxation techniques, some of which employ a methodical contraction and relaxation of the muscles of various parts of the body, and some which call for focusing attention on various parts of the body while employing autosuggestion to induce warm sensations, heaviness, and a feeling of serenity. Various meditation and biofeedback techniques also help in muscle relaxation. It is almost certain, however, that the most important factor in the lack of normal sleep is not related to the muscles at all but to the way the patient thinks. Apart from muscle relaxation, the common factor in all these methods of treatment is the diversion of attention from thoughts that bother us to more pleasant and monotonous internal feelings. "Merciful powers, restrain me in the cursed thoughts that nature gives way to in repose!" pleads Banquo in *Macbeth*. The curbing of thoughts is almost certainly the key to falling asleep. This idea is the basis of the oldest method of all—counting sheep. There is no doubt that thought arousal is one of the commonest symptoms in insomniacs. It is difficult to fall asleep when you are constantly turning over in your mind the causes of your disagreement with your business partner, whether or not to buy some stocks, or the reason for failing an important examination. It is also difficult to fall asleep if you are lying in bed fearing "yet another sleepless night."

As not all insomnia sufferers are necessarily tense, the various relaxation techniques must be adapted to the subject's needs. The condition of insomniacs who get into bed serene and relaxed can be worsened by the use of relaxation techniques. To obtain the maximum benefit from the various techniques, thirty minutes of daily practice is essential. This should start during the day; only once the required level of proficiency has been attained should the techniques be practiced before going to bed.

## SLEEP HYGIENE

Apart from therapeutic methods designed to prepare for sleep, insomniacs should observe a number of simple behavioral rules that will help them adapt to correct sleeping habits. Surprisingly enough, the adoption of good habits can be of greater help than any other therapeutic technique.

1. Do not spend too much time in bed. Limit the time you spend in bed to sleeping. If you have woken up, get out of bed. Go back to bed only when you are ready to sleep.

2. Do not try to force yourself to sleep. The more you try to fall asleep, the more your arousal level will increase and sleep will be impossible. Generations of insomniacs have counted sheep in order to avoid thinking about sleep. If you tend to fall asleep in front of the television yet find it difficult to do so in bed, try watching television in bed and fit a time clock to the set that will switch it off about an hour after you have fallen asleep.

3. Get rid of the clock in your bedroom; its ticking and luminous dial can easily prevent even people who do not suffer from insomnia from falling asleep.

4. Avoid physical activity in the late evening hours. One of the commonest misconceptions among insomniacs is that of the benefits of strenuous physical activity just before going to bed. Remember, physical activity raises the level of arousal. There are, of course, benefits to be reaped from regular exercise, but it should be done at least two hours before going to bed.

5. Avoid drinking coffee and alcohol and smoking before going to bed. I have often met people who claimed that coffee didn't affect them at all; on the contrary, they couldn't fall asleep without drinking a cup of coffee. I am sorry to have to disappoint coffee addicts, but caffeine, like nicotine, is a stimulant that causes awakening. The reason that people who are used to drinking coffee do not feel its effects immediately is that it is not the caffeine itself that stimulates but the products of its breaking down. Therefore, the effects of coffee begin to be felt only about

an hour after it has been drunk. I have also heard people say that alcohol has no effect on sleep. But worse than that are the many people who have told me that they use it to treat insomnia. Alcohol does produce a feeling of drowsiness, so the person who has a glass of brandy or vodka before going to bed feels slightly drowsy and ready to go to sleep. But once the alcohol has broken down in the body, the compounds released have a stimulating effect, and so many people who use alcohol to help them fall asleep find themselves awake in the middle of the night and unable to fall asleep again.

6. Go to sleep and wake up at regular hours. A routine in bed-time and waking-up hours is of great importance. Many people have no difficulty falling asleep even if they get into bed at a different hour every day, but for sufferers from insomnia, irregular sleeping and waking hours may worsen the condition. A good example of this is "Sunday night insomnia," which is a popular complaint even among those who do not suffer from chronic insomnia. Its sufferers have usually been partying on Saturday night until the early hours of Sunday morning. Then they sleep until lunchtime and as a result have difficulty falling asleep on Sunday night. Waking up on Monday morning for a new working week presents, of course, a big problem.

7. Do not eat a heavy meal before going to bed. Carbohydrates and protein are recommended, but not chocolate or large amounts of sugars. Do not drink any beverage excessively before going to bed. If you do wake up in the middle of the night, don't make for the refrigerator—it could become a habit!

8. Do not sleep during the day. That does not mean that there is anything wrong with a siesta, but the luxury of an afternoon sleep for insomniacs is likely to exacerbate an already severe condition. Staying awake during the day increases the need to sleep at night, thus making falling asleep that much easier.

## SLEEPING DRUGS

Drugs for sleeping were among the first to be used by humans. Hypnos, the ancient Greek god of sleep, is depicted in bas-reliefs carrying a sheaf of poppies, the seeds of which were used to prepare the first sleeping drugs. During the Middle Ages, when the ladies of the court had difficulty sleeping, they would suck on a swab that had been dipped into a "cock-tail" of poppy juice and alcohol. Ancient medical books tell us that numerous plants were used in sleeping drafts, from chamomile flowers to lettuce. Mention of this was the cause of a minor sensation in one of my lectures. At a medical seminar on sleep disorders, I made a humorous reference to the use of lettuce as a sleeping drug and recommended that my audience begin writing prescriptions for "three or four lettuce leaves instead of a sleeping pill." I had no idea that the gist of my lecture had been given to the press. My "recommendation" about lettuce was taken in all seriousness and received prominent coverage in one of the more popular Israeli papers. Next day, the telephones in the Sleep Laboratory did not stop ringing. Scores if not hundreds of people called to obtain a prescription for "sleeping lettuce." Even the publication of a letter to the paper's editor which stated categorically that "lettuce is only lettuce" had no effect. The lettuce story spread like wildfire, and one woman even called the laboratory to complain that she was suffering from stomach poisoning after eating a large portion of lettuce before going to sleep! Humorous as it is, the incident gives an indication of the large number of people who need sleeping drugs and who are willing to try anything to improve their sleep.

There is no exact information regarding the number of people who use sleeping drugs regularly. The accepted assumption is that 5–8 percent of the adult population of the Western countries use them several times a week. It is also accepted knowledge that the use of sleeping drugs increases with age and that women use them more than men.

The most common sleeping drugs are from the benzodiazepine family and are sold under a variety of proprietary names. The extensive use of drugs from this family began at the end of the 1960s. Until that time, the most popular sleeping drugs were from the barbiturate family, which were introduced around the turn of the century. The best known were amobarbital (Amytal), secobarbital (Seconal), and pentobarbital (Nembutal).

Then the first scientific studies of sleep delivered a telling blow to the use of barbiturates. Tests on barbiturate users in the sleep laboratory showed that the drugs caused undesirable changes in sleep structure, depressing REM sleep and the deep sleep of stages 3 and 4. Moreover, chronic barbiturate users who had taken the drugs for months and even years slept worse with the help of the drugs than without it. The publication of these findings, and the appearance on the market of new drugs from the benzodiazepine family, ended the use of barbiturates as a treatment for insomnia. The pharmaceutical companies invested huge sums in the development and testing of new drugs in sleep laboratories, and later in advertising campaigns based on laboratory findings. The investment sunk into the development of each new drug could be as high as tens of millions of dollars.

I was an eyewitness to this type of no-holds-barred competition at the start of my career as a sleep researcher, as my postdoctoral studies at the University of San Diego Sleep Laboratory were financed by a pharmaceutical company. In return for the grant, I had to test the effects of a certain drug on chronic insomniacs. I studied the structure of their sleep as determined by electrophysiological recordings in the laboratory and recorded their subjective feelings about the drug after they had woken up in the morning.

At the conclusion of the study, a representative of the company came to interview me. The meeting was somewhat strange: instead of asking me about the sleep laboratory findings regarding the efficacy of the drug, she was interested only in its side effects. The subjects had indeed complained of bothersome side effects, such as headaches and impaired concentration and memory after awakening. The company's representative urged me to give her complete details of any possible side effects but showed no interest at all in the drug's efficacy in the treatment of sleep disorders. Bewildered, I went to see the head of our laboratory, Dan Kripke, and expressed surprise that the company had invested so much money only in order to investigate the side effects of its drugs. He looked at me incredulously and replied, "I can't believe that you're so naive. Do you really think they manufacture the drug themselves?" Only then did I realize, much to my amazement, that the pharmaceutical company financed my study in order to test a product of a rival company. My findings about side effects were presented to the United States Food and Drug

Administration to prove that the harm caused by the drug was greater than its benefits. I do not know whether my study had anything to do with it, but use of that particular drug was stopped some years later.

Sleeping drugs can provide an efficient solution for sleep disorder, but the choice of a suitable drug is of paramount importance. There are considerable differences between the various drugs, the principal one being in the speed of absorption and the length of the drug's half-life. The majority of drugs on the market today are absorbed relatively rapidly and take effect within twenty to forty-five minutes. But the duration of their efficacy varies significantly. This duration is measured by the drug's half-life—the time required for the level of the substance to decrease to one-half of its maximum level in the blood, at a specific dosage. The level of the substance in the bloodstream drops as it is absorbed by the body's tissues and removed by the liver. The half-life of sleeping drugs on the market today varies from one to eighty hours or more.

The longer the half-life of the drug, the greater the risk that it will have undesirable residual effects on both the level of alertness and the following day's functional level. People who take a sleeping drug with a half-life that exceeds twelve hours will awake with the drug level in their blood still high, and this will affect their functioning—particularly their level of alertness—throughout the day. Many people who take sleeping drugs with a long half-life complain of waking up confused and tired. Their reactions are slow. These symptoms take several hours to dissipate, if they do at all.

A further disadvantage of sleeping drugs with a long half-life is that they tend to accumulate in the body. When people take a sleeping drug with a half-life longer than twenty-four hours every day for several consecutive days, the drug level in their bloodstream will rise each day, even if the dosage remains the same. Therefore, after a few days, the true dosage is likely to be much higher than that prescribed by the doctor. This will increase the residual effects of the drug during the day. However, it is worth noting that drugs with a long half-life are advantageous in cases that require tranquilization of the patient during the day.

Sleeping drugs with a short half-life of up to two hours can have equally undesirable effects. As the level of the drug in the blood drops so rapidly, the drug loses its effectiveness half-way through sleep. The sleeper will awaken in the middle of the night and find it difficult to fall asleep again. For this reason, such drugs are unsuitable for those who suffer from frequent awakenings and should be prescribed only for people who have difficulty falling asleep.

In light of the undesirable effects of sleeping drugs that have a very long or a very short half-life, there is a clear advantage to using sleeping drugs that have an average half-life of four to six hours. The use of these drugs ensures an effectiveness level in the blood that will be maintained throughout the night, but without any residual effects the following day.

But even people who take the sleeping drug ideally suited to their condition must adhere to three basic rules in order to ensure that the drug has the optimal effect and does not paradoxically worsen the insomnia. The first rule concerns when to take the sleeping drug. Many people who take such drugs view it as a sign of weakness, an admission that they are unable to deal with sleep disorders unaided. So every night they wrestle with whether to take a sleeping pill or to try to fall asleep without its help. In many cases, the decision is a compromise: they do without a pill and "see what happens." If they manage to fall asleep without the pill, well and good. If not, they reconcile themselves to their weakness and take the pill one hour, two hours, or even three hours later. So, having despaired of falling asleep unaided, they take their "life-saving" pill at 3 A.M. I can readily understand the inner struggle of insomniacs and even appreciate their efforts to face their sleeping problems without the aid of drugs. But if confronting the problem means postponing the taking of a sleeping pill, then the sleep disorder could further deteriorate.

When a person gets into bed after having made a firm decision to fall asleep whatever happens, the decision itself is the cause of tension and anxiety which act as a stimulant. As I mentioned earlier, sleep must come of its own volition; we have no means of forcing it. Frequent glances at the bedside clock to check whether it is time to take the sleeping pill are a tried and tested recipe for a sleepless night. Moreover, once the fateful decision has been made and the pill is finally taken in the early hours of the morning, the risk of undesirable side effects during the day is greatly increased. A person who takes a sleeping pill at 3 or 4 A.M. and wakes up at 7 A.M. in order to get to work on time will still be under the influence of the drug, even if it has a short half-life. This can have a serious effect on the person's functional level, especially in activities that call for a high level of alertness, like driving.

Sleeping drugs must therefore be taken according to a preset plan, and not according to a feeling that varies from night to night. Bedtime should be predetermined and the pill taken some twenty to thirty minutes beforehand. This rule should be observed throughout the treatment.

The second rule concerns the effective range of sleeping drugs. How long can one take a sleeping drug continuously? Sleep laboratory studies have shown that the effective range of the majority of sleeping drugs is limited to two to three weeks. Once this period is up, tolerance is created and the drug, at best, ceases to have any effect; at worst, it exacerbates the sleep disorder. To extend the effective range of the drug, its use should be interrupted for three or four days after the initial two to three weeks and then resumed at the same dosage. During the interval, the disorder may return or even worsen. In any event, even when it is clear that the drug is having no further effect, the dosage must not be increased or another drug added without consulting a doctor. To encourage the insomnia patient to use sleeping drugs correctly, we usually tell them that they are signing a contract with the drug, as it were: the drug undertakes to improve their sleep, while they undertake to observe the rules of use strictly. Any deviation from the rules is just cause for "breach of contract" and a good reason for terminating the use of the drug.

The third rule concerns stopping the prolonged use of sleeping drugs, which creates both tolerance to and dependency on the drugs. It is important to emphasize that mental dependency on a drug bears no relation to its efficacy. People who have developed a dependency on sleeping drugs would not consider going to bed without them, even when it is clear beyond doubt that drugs do not help them sleep. Withdrawal in cases like this is often as difficult as withdrawal from alcohol use, or even from the use of hard drugs. During the withdrawal period, the patient suffers from severe sleep disorders, frightening dreams and nightmares, and heightened anxiety during the day. After a day or two without sleep, many people throw in the towel and go back to using sleeping drugs, usually at an increased dosage. I described this earlier as one way in which temporary insomnia is turned into chronic insomnia. People like this are usually unable to withdraw completely from sleeping drug use without hospitalization. To help patients withdraw completely, the use of sleeping drugs must be stopped gradually. The dosage is slowly decreased in controlled stages. In most cases, the quality of the patients' sleep at the end of the withdrawal period is higher than that of their drug-assisted sleep.

# The Physical and Medical Causes of Insomnia

A minority of insomniacs suffer from some physical problem, principally periodic leg movements and respiratory disorders. The latter, which are mostly associated with excessive sleepiness but may be also linked to insomnia, will be discussed in greater detail in Chapter 19.

Ten percent of the insomnia patients referred to the Technion Sleep Laboratory suffer from periodic leg movements during sleep. Similar observations have been reported by other sleep clinics. In this condition, the patients' legs move every fifteen to twenty seconds while they are asleep. The movements may be small—limited to one foot or just the toes—or they may involve the entire leg. Some cause brief or long awakenings. The number of movements per night, ranging from one hundred to five hundred, determines the severity of the syndrome. Typical complaints of patients who suffer from this condition are frequent awakenings for no apparent reason and morning fatigue. Some complain about their legs—muscle cramps after awakening, pains in the legs, or stiff muscles. A small number of patients complain of leg discomfort while sitting or lying down, forcing them to walk around in order to get relief. This disorder is called "nervous legs syndrome," and almost all those who suffer from it have periodic leg movements during sleep.

Periodic leg movements are common among diabetics, patients who suffer from kidney disease and who are undergoing dialysis, and those who suffer from rheumatic ailments. The patients' ages are generally higher than those of patients who suffer from situational or chronic insomnia, or patients who have a background of mental disorder. Patients who suffer from periodic leg movements during sleep do not usually respond to treatment with sleeping drugs. The most efficient treatment found so far is clonazepam, a drug usually given to epileptic children. As tolerance to this drug can be created after prolonged use, it should be used with the same circumspection as sleeping drugs.

Insomnia may also accompany a large number of medical disorders. In these conditions, although insomnia is not the primary problem, the difficulty of obtaining a restful sleep can exacerbate the underlying medical condition. Impairment of sleep has been described in patients with head injuries and in those with various pains, including headaches. Cancer patients in particular, who frequently suffer from chronic pain, complain about insomnia more than other medical or surgical patients. It is possible, however, that emotional factors also play a role in these patients.

Among hospitalized patients, the intensive care unit is undoubtedly the environment most hostile to sleep. Several researchers monitored the sleep of patients in intensive care units during the first few days after their operations. In many cases it appeared that during the first couple of days after a major operation, patients hardly slept at all. The noise of the machines and staff activity, the bright light, and patients' pain added up to a sure recipe for sleepless nights. This situation must be changed if we truly believe that sleep is important for patients' recuperation.

Sleep studies of patients in chronic pain also revealed a unique pattern of brain waves during sleep: the alpha-delta sleep pattern. When these patients are in the deep sleep of stages 3 and 4, instead of high-amplitude delta activity, they have a mixture of alpha activity—which indicates wakefulness—and delta waves. It appears that the brain centers regulating wakefulness and sleep are activated simultaneously. Thus, although alpha-delta sleep has been associated with a variety of medical conditions, such as chronic pain, rheumatoid arthritis, and post-traumatic recovery, there is a common thread to patients' complaints: they all complained about nonrestorative sleep, chronic fatigue, and malaise. It is also no wonder that these patients describe their sleep as light and fragmented.

Whenever sleep accompanies a medical disorder, treatment should be directed first and foremost at the underlying disease. Supportive treatment for the sleep disorders should be attempted whenever the quality of sleep is so poor that it affects patients' condition and behavior.

## INSOMNIA AND MENTAL DISORDERS

Severe sleep disorders are also part of the clinical picture in many cases of mental disturbance. In mental disorder syndromes that result from dementia, for example, sleep disorders are another aspect of patients' overall agitation. They are likely to awaken confused and disoriented, and sometimes behave automatically—for example, sleepwalking. In a study conducted at the Technion Sleep Laboratory on acutely demented patients, we found that the majority suffered from sleep disorders in both the continuity of their sleep and its timing. It is not entirely impossible that these sleep disorders are caused by degeneration of the brain centers which control sleep and its regularity, or of the nerve pathways leading to them.

Severe sleep disorders are typical in patients suffering from schizophrenia or other psychoses. Difficulty in falling asleep and frequent awakenings are likely to develop as a result of anxiety combined with patients' heightened suspicions, guilt feelings, or dysfunctional thought processes. Patients are sometimes frightened to sleep because of delusions that something terrible is likely to happen to them. Sometimes turbulent thoughts by day and night prevent falling asleep: the degree of sleep disturbances parallels the severity of the psychiatric symptoms. No typical symptoms of the sleep of psychotic patients have been found in studies conducted in sleep laboratories, but some reports indicate that schizophrenic patients may have shortened REM latencies, as depressed patients do, and that about half of them have reduced deep sleep. In almost all cases, the sleep disorder was not the predominant complaint of the psychotic patient, but medical literature documents psychotic crises which occurred after a period of acute insomnia. In other words, the lack of sleep prepared the ground, as it were, for the mental crisis. Therefore, great attention should be paid to severe sleep difficulties that suddenly appear in young people, especially when they are accompanied by complaints of severe anxiety for no reason, dysfunction of the thought processes, or frightening hallucinations.

The only mental illness in which there are characteristic complaints regarding sleep, and in which the patients' sleep patterns show unique markers, is depression. It is rare to encounter patients with a mood disorder who do not have disrupted sleep-wakefulness cycles, and the majority complain of insomnia. The two forms of depression in which sleep has been extensively studied are major and bipolar depression. The latter is characterized by a succession of depressive and manic episodes in which the patient suddenly shifts from severe depression to extreme hyperactivity. Common to all the forms of depression are moodiness, loss of interest in what is going on, and a lack of ability to feel enjoyment or pleasure. Additional symptoms are loss of appetite, fatigue, restlessness, feelings of guilt and low self-esteem, and difficulty in concentration. Thoughts of suicide—and even suicide attempts—are not rare. The incidence of disturbed sleep in depression is so high that it also serves as a diagnostic symptom.

The sleep recordings of depressive patients show a number of characteristic variations, most prominently in REM sleep latency. REM sleep, which in normal people appears some seventy to ninety minutes after falling asleep, appears in depressive patients after only thirty to forty minutes, and sometimes even sooner. Furthermore, the duration of the first REM sleep in depressive patients is longer and more turbulent than in normal people; in other words, it is characterized by high density of eye movements. Depressed patients also show greatly reduced deep sleep and tend to awake in midsleep and be unable to reinitiate sleep. The identification of these variations on the sleep recording sometimes helps in the diagnosis of the depression itself, as the following example shows.

An obese hospital nurse, with a short thick neck, came to the Sleep Laboratory complaining of tiredness and fatigue during the day, and frequent awakenings at night. She also complained of loud snoring and tiredness upon awakening. All these symptoms raised the possibility that she was suffering from sleep apnea, but this diagnosis was rejected because there was no evidence of respiratory disorders. (Sleep apnea will be discussed in detail in Chapter 19.) The most prominent finding in the sleep recording was the appearance of the first REM sleep some twenty minutes after the patient had fallen asleep. It continued for more than fifteen minutes and was unusually turbulent. When I met the nurse to discuss our findings, my first question was whether she had noticed any change in her mood over the past few weeks. I had hardly got the words out of my mouth when she burst into heart-rending tears. In great agitation, she told me that for many years her mother had suffered from severe depression which had required treatment and hospitalization. She feared that she too was suffering from the illness. Instead of seeking medical advice, she had simply denied the possibility and convinced herself that changes in her behavior were caused by respiratory problems during sleep. Treatment with antidepressants brought about a marked improvement in her condition, and the sleep disorders disappeared.

Indeed, in all cases of sleep disorders that are accompanied by mental disturbance, treatment must be directed first and foremost at the mental disorder. Although supporting treatment of the sleep disorder is sometimes required, an improvement in sleep will not occur before the patient's mental condition has been improved.

# Disorders in Sleep Timing

In the chapter on sleep-wakefulness rhythms, I described a student whose sleep-wakefulness rhythm was longer than twenty-four hours and who, as a result, could not maintain a "normal" daily schedule. That case demonstrates one possible disorder in sleep timing: the biological clock works independently of the external environment, and so the patient goes to sleep later and later every day. Although this disorder is extremely rare, such cases indicate that normal sleep demands precise coordination between the biological clock that controls sleep and the environmental clock. When this coordination is disrupted and the environmental light-dark cycle no longer entrains the daily deviation of the endogenous biological clock, the life of these patients is plunged into chaos. So long as the clock dictates that they sleep at night, they manage to maintain a normal schedule. But after a few days, when the clock dictates that they sleep during the day, their schedule is upset and goes out of control. If the duration of their cycle were to be lengthened permanently—say, to twenty-five hours—so that their sleep underwent a fixed daily delay of one hour, then it might be possible to plan a schedule around their "personal" clock. For example, they might be able to make important appointments only on those days of the month in which the wakefulness hours corresponded to the daytime hours. But the majority of people who suffer from this disorder do not have a permanent sleep-wakefulness cycle; furthermore, it may change suddenly every few days for no apparent reason. This, of course, obviates any possibility of planning a schedule.

A total loss of coordination between the external environment and the biological clock is extremely rare. Of the more than fifteen thousand people who have been examined at the Technion Sleep Laboratory, only a few had sleep-wakefulness rhythms longer than twenty-four hours. Two were blind persons, which is hardly surprising, for sleep timing disorders are particularly common among the blind. As we have already seen, alternating environmental light and darkness is the most significant factor that causes the biological clock to conform to the geophysical day. Losing the ability to experience the changes of light and darkness is likely to force the biological clock "escape" from the constraints of environmental rhythms.

The most common of all sleep timing disorders is a permanent deviation of the sleep phase relative to the geophysical day. People who suffer from this disorder are radical and uncompromising "night owls." The sleeping habits of the majority of night creatures are not usually a hindrance, but once the coordination between the biological clock and the environment is lost, the sleep disorder causes severe functional disorder. The most conspicuous sign of delayed sleep phase syndrome, as it is known in scientific literature, is in the way patients describe their complaint. They say they are unable to fall asleep earlier than the small hours of the night; once they do fall asleep, they continue undisturbed but are unable to wake up before about noon. Unlike patients who suffer from situational or chronic insomnia and who can be helped with sleeping drugs, cases of delayed sleep are not treatable by medication. The only way to combat this sleep disorder is to wait patiently for the opening of the "sleep gate" that often occurs only at sunrise.

As of this writing, we have tested more than one hundred people who have come to the Sleep Laboratory suffering from delayed sleep phase syndrome. We found several factors which were common to many of them. Some tried to combat their disorder by looking for an occupation that would allow them to live a normal life as night owls. One of the women patients, for example, owned a bar that remained open until the early hours of the morning. Another patient had always worked night shifts and slept during the day. Their problem became acute once they retired and wanted to wake up in the morning, just like everyone else. Indeed, one of the most serious complaints heard from the majority of these patients—sometimes even more serious than the problem of falling asleep—was their difficulty in waking up at a normally accepted hour. People who are unable to wake up before 4 P.M. will find it hard to function in a society in which the normal working day begins at 8 or 9 A.M. and finishes at 5 P.M.

Another factor common to delayed sleep phase syndrome sufferers is the age at which the disorder first makes its appearance. Patients report that they have "always" had their falling-asleep and awakening difficulties. Some claim that they remember experiencing difficulty in falling asleep as children. In some cases, parents and other family members confirmed these recollections. One mother described going for walks with her three-year-old son at the "strange hours" of 1 and 2 A.M.; she had been unable to get him to sleep before 3 A.M. But her main problem had been the suspicious glances of her neighbors!

As a rule, the people diagnosed as suffering from delayed sleep phase syndrome were younger than those who suffered from insomnia and had a background of mental disturbance. Before they reached the Sleep Laboratory, many of them had tried all kinds of different treatments, usually without much success. Another common factor is that some of these patients suffered from a behavioral disturbance that called for psychiatric treatment. In our view, in some cases at least, the behavioral disturbance had its roots in the sleep disorder. People whose sleeping hours have been completely opposite to those around them from a very early age, and whose efforts to change this situation have been doomed to failure, are in a permanent state of frustration. Such a situation was described beautifully by one of our young patients. He told us that as a punishment for never getting to school in time for the first period, he had had to report to the principal's office half an hour earlier—which was, of course, impossible for him. From there, the road to expulsion from school had been short, and he was transferred to a special education facility. That young man, whom the army refused to enlist because of sleep and behavioral disorders, was treated with great success in our laboratory. Within a few months, he managed to make up the ground he had lost at school and was inducted into the army. His successful integration into the military was extremely gratifying to us.

We have no data on the exact number of delayed sleep phase syndrome sufferers, but the lack of public awareness of the syndrome dooms them all to a frustrating conflict with society. Those who fall asleep the moment their head touches the pillow find it difficult to comprehend that there are people who cannot wake up on time or fall asleep. I have come across this self-centered attitude time and again in the Sleep Laboratory when I have been asked to counsel married couples. In most cases, the woman suffers from insomnia and her husband asks us to explain to her that "she only thinks she suffers from sleeplessness." He then goes on to give reasons for his "diagnosis": "It simply isn't possible that someone who really wants to sleep cannot do so." It is therefore easy to understand the frustration of parents whose child is unable to wake up on time for school but is not prepared to go to bed before the small hours of the night. In nearly every case, the explanation of such "strange" behavior is the child's attitude to studies, parents, or life in general. Imposing punishments and demanding that the child wake up on time at any price usually only serves to exacerbate the problem and divert it to psychiatric treatment with its concomitant stigma, from which it is almost impossible to escape later in life.

It is therefore recommended that attention be paid, from an early age, to any deviation in the sleep habits of children. If there is difficulty in their waking up in the morning, and difficulty in falling asleep before the early hours of the morning, it should not be put down to childish capriciousness, laziness, or rebelliousness. The child should be examined for the possibility of the existence of a sleep disorder. Expecting everyone to wake up at 6 A.M. feeling refreshed and ready to greet the morning with a smile is about as logical as telling them to sleep for eight hours precisely and not a minute less. Our experience over the past two years has shown us that the first people who should bear in mind the existence of delayed sleep phase syndrome are primary and high school principals and teachers. Children who experience chronic problems waking up in the morning may have a body clock that is not adjusted to their environmental demands.

And what about the advanced sleep phase syndrome—in other words, a deviation in the coordination between the biological clock and the alternation of night and day that advances the sleep phase? It might be expected that the advanced sleep phase syndrome would be as common as its delayed counterpart, but that is not so. So far, I have encountered very few cases of this type of sleep timing disorder. These people came to the Sleep Laboratory with a similar complaint: they had to go to bed in the early hours of the evening, around 7 P.M., and woke up refreshed and ready to face the day "in the middle of the night"—at 2 or 3 A.M.—after having slept for seven or eight hours. One of them did not even request treatment; he had come merely to obtain official medical verification that he was not suffering from any kind of mental disturbance. He requested this in writing for his wife, who refused to accept his strange sleep habits. Most important, his advanced sleep phase was affecting their social life, as he was unable to stay awake at any of the gatherings they attended. In another case, a woman in her forties came to the Sleep Laboratory as a result of the tension that had arisen between her and her husband because of her unusual sleep habits. In this case, the conflict was so serious that we did try to bring about a change.

We have no convincing explanation of why the number of those who suffer from advanced sleep phase syndrome is so small, but as we have seen, the natural tendency of the biological clock is to delay the time of sleep, not to advance it. It is therefore a reasonable assumption that if the coordination between the biological clock and the external environment is disrupted, it will result in the delay of sleep and not in its advance. As we shall see, this characteristic has been put to good therapeutic use.

## CHRONOTHERAPY OR PHOTOTHERAPY?

The late Elliot Weitzman of the Montefiore Hospital in New York, one of the pillars of the pioneering group of sleep researchers, was the first to apply the principles of the biological clock which controls sleep and wakefulness to the treatment of delayed sleep phase syndrome. The principal reason for the inability of those who suffer from the syndrome to advance their sleep, claimed Weitzman, was that it was opposed to the natural tendency of the biological clock to delay the time for sleep. Weitzman and his colleagues proposed treating delayed sleep phase syndrome sufferers by a controlled delay of their sleeping hours until they reached the desired sleeping time. Thus, a person who went to bed around midnight and found it difficult to fall asleep before 4 A.M. would delay bedtime until 8 A.M. for two or three days. Then it would be pushed back to noon, 4 P.M., 8 P.M., and finally midnight. Weitzman and his colleagues predicted that the patients would not encounter any particular difficulty in this delay of their sleep, and that after a few days they would go to sleep at the desired time.

The technique worked. Delayed sleep phase syndrome sufferers can easily delay their sleep from day to day and then stop once they have reached the sleeping time that suits them. There is, however, one small problem. The treatment, which must be carried out gradually, requires total dedication of the subject to sleep at precisely predetermined times for a month or more. Some of these times occur in the middle of the day, which may interfere with work and family life. The treatment also demands commitment and strict adherence to the preferred sleeping time once it has been achieved. Any deviation from this hour may result in the "escape" of sleep once more. Although the results of the treatment are usually good, many people are simply unable to contend with its demands.

The therapeutic approach to delayed sleep phase syndrome changed significantly with the discovery that bright light at an intensity of at least 2,500 lux affects the sleep-wakefulness clock and depresses the secretion of melatonin. In order to advance the sleep phase by a few hours—say, from 4 A.M. to midnight—subjects should be exposed to bright light during the morning. To delay sleeping time from, say, 8 P.M. to midnight, they should be exposed to the bright light during the evening. Treatment with bright light in order to readjust the biological clock has proved to be extremely efficient. Several days after patients have been exposed to the light, a shift in their sleeping hours is usually observed. The shift is usually gradual, and two to three weeks of exposure to light are required in order to achieve the desired change in sleeping times.

Light treatment is performed using a special high-intensity lamp, or by exposure to sunlight—which we used with great success during the summer months. As we had discovered in one of our studies on blind people that their sleep disorders were linked to a disruption of the melatonin secretion rhythm, we have recently begun to use melatonin in the treatment of sleep timing disorders in sighted patients. Our first findings showed that when melatonin was administered at the correct time, it forced the "sleep gate" into a day/night cycle.

## "THE CLOCK'S WRONG": HUMAN INTERVENTION

For tens of thousands of years, the setting sun was the signal for human beings to find shelter for the night, and sunrise told them that night was over and they could emerge. The invention of the electric light bulb by Edison—who, according to popular legend, hardly slept at all—and the rapid spread of artificial light freed us from the shackles of sunrise and sunset. Since then, modern society has been characterized by "life around the clock." There are industries and services which do not stop working even for a minute.

Night work obliges us to move our sleep to the daytime hours either permanently or on alternate weeks or months. The usual way of filling jobs that demand around-the-clock work is by shift work. The workers are organized into three shifts of seven or eight hours each, usually designated "morning," "evening," and "night." The composition of the shifts varies from place to place and from plant to plant, according to local tradition and the type of plant. What, then, is the difference between sleep during the day after a night shift and sleep during the night after a day shift? Many studies have shown that sleep during the day is shorter by about two hours than sleep during the night, even in ideal conditions. The reason for this is to be found in the sleeping time in accordance with the body temperature curve. It will be remembered that the body temperature curve reaches its lowest daily point during the early hours of the morning, and its highest daily point during the evening. Unlike the daytime worker who goes to sleep when the curve is descending, the night worker goes to bed when the body temperature curve is in the ascendant. As in the isolation studies described in chapter 5, the periods of sleep when the body temperature curve is rising were shorter than those when it was dropping. Furthermore, sleeping conditions in many workers' homes are far from ideal—bedrooms cannot be sealed to prevent the intrusion of noise and sunlight. We can therefore easily understand why sleep disorders are so common among shift workers, and this is one of the main reasons for the adjustment difficulties that are part of working alternating shifts.

In the past few years, the Technion Sleep Laboratory has conducted an extensive study of shift work. We tried to discover whether it was possible to improve adjustment to alternating shifts by improved planning of sleep hours, and whether it was possible to determine workers' suitability to alternate shift work by evaluating the quality of their sleep, among other things. As sleep in the sleep laboratory does not accurately reflect sleep in the worker's home, this study required the use of moni-

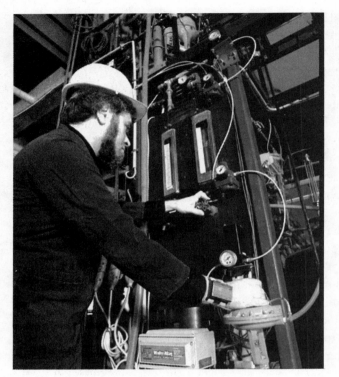

Fig. 30. Study on
the sleep of shift
workers: the acti-
meter is on the
right wrist.

toring techniques in the home. We used a computerized actimeter which
was worn on the worker's wrist and which recorded all hand movements
and stored them in its memory. The metered data were later transferred
to a computer for processing and the identification of periods of sleep
and wakefulness.

Figure 31 shows a day worker's recording, while in figure 32 we can
see the sleep-wakefulness rhythm of a shift worker at a plant with the
three-shift system. The shifts commence on Sundays and finish on Thurs-
days, with Fridays and Saturdays free. The big variation that occurs at
the sleeping time of each shift can be seen clearly. In this study, too,
when the sleep and wakefulness recordings were made at the workers'
homes, we discovered that sleep during the day was shorter than that at
night—some five hours compared to approximately seven. We also discovered that many shift workers tended to split their daytime sleep into

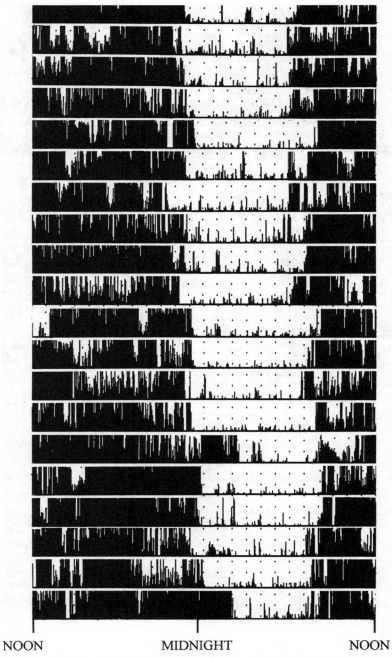

DAYS

NOON       MIDNIGHT       NOON

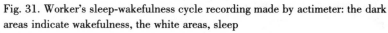

Fig. 31. Worker's sleep-wakefulness cycle recording made by actimeter: the dark areas indicate wakefulness, the white areas, sleep

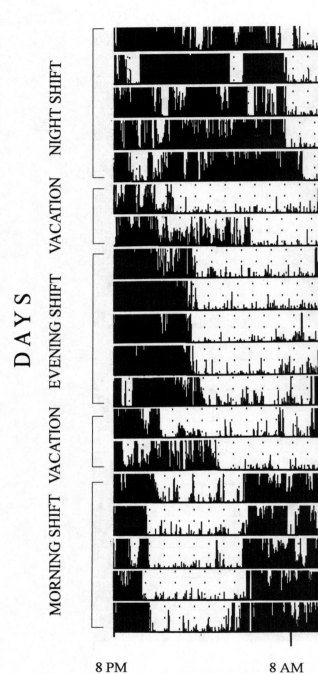

Fig. 32. Shift worker's sleep-wakefulness cycle when shift rotates: night, evening, morning

two or more parts, sleeping once during the morning and then again during the afternoon.

Is it possible to enhance workers' adjustability by planning the shifts in a way that accommodates the biological clock which controls sleep and wakefulness? Several factors should be taken into account. The shift rota, or the number of consecutive days the worker spends on each shift, is of the utmost significance. The "slower" rotas popular in the United States change shifts every two to four weeks, while the "faster" ones in use especially in Japan and Europe change every three to five days. Both systems have their advantages and disadvantages. The theoretical advantage of the slow rota is in better adjustment of the circadian rhythms to the night shift. As the adaptation period is usually seven to ten days, it may be assumed that at its conclusion the worker is at the optimal adjustment stage. But a number of studies have shown that adjustment to night work is not complete even after two or three weeks. On their days off, workers prefer to change over from daytime to nighttime sleep, so that in fact their night shifts are not of several consecutive weeks. This is the reason for the extension of the adjustment period. In the fast rota, there is no real change in the circadian rhythms; they remain coordinated with environmental rhythms, and this is the advantage of this rota system. Some researchers assume that maintaining the coordination between the body's rhythms and those of the environment contributes to the worker's adjustment and in the long term prevents damage to his health.

The direction of the shift rota is also very important. The shift rota system can be operated "clockwise" (morning-evening-night) or "counterclockwise" (night-evening-morning). Given the choice, many workers prefer the counterclockwise direction because they gain a long weekend when they change from the night to the evening shift. Now that we are aware of the inclination of the biological clock when free from environmental constraints to delay sleep from day to day, we should clearly prefer the clockwise rota, because under it sleep comes later from shift to shift.

Awareness of the special situation of shift workers, resulting from the perpetual change their bodily clocks undergo, has increased immeasurably in recent years. One of the main reasons for this heightened awareness is the ever-increasing price that society has to pay for human error and industrial accidents. In the nineteenth century, the only people who worked at night were gatekeepers, cooks, and, according to some historical evidence, the court tailors, especially before state banquets and galas. Today, the fate of millions is in the hands of the night shift workers at nuclear facilities and power stations. The accident at the Chernobyl nuclear facility in the former Soviet Union apparently occurred as a result of a series of errors made by its operators at 2 A.M., during the night shift. We were only a hairsbreadth away from an ecological holocaust of unimaginable proportions. The accidents at the Three Mile Island nuclear facility in the United States and the Union Carbide factory at Bhopal, India, also occurred in the early morning. The horrifying possibility that a sleepy night shift worker might press the wrong button and cause radioactive contamination of vast dimensions dictates a different approach to the people who have to remain awake while the rest of the world sleeps.

## JET LAG

In an age in which manned space ships circle above us and millions of people use intercontinental flights every year, the phenomenon known as "jet lag" has become a matter of routine. Everyone knows that in the first few days after a flight from Israel to the United States or in the reverse direction, we suffer from sleeping difficulties at night and from drowsiness and fatigue during the day. Some people suffer these symptoms for only a day or two, while others recover fully only after a week or more. Like shift work, we can view jet lag as part of the price that humankind has to pay for technological progress. The direct cause of jet lag is the limited capability of the body's clocks to keep up with rapid changes in the environmental clocks.

To demonstrate this, let us join a businessman who is booked on a direct flight from Tel Aviv to New York. Our companion arrived at Ben Gurion Airport in Tel Aviv at 6 A.M., refreshed after seven hours of sleep in his own bed. After takeoff at 8 A.M., he relaxed in his business-class seat and, after having breakfast, busied himself with the pile of documents on the table before him. At 2 P.M., six hours after takeoff and high over the British Isles, he partook of a lavish lunch that included a vintage wine. The wine made him a little sleepy, so he pressed a button, adjusted his seat to the reclining position, drew the window blind, covered his eyes with a sleep mask which had thoughtfully been provided by a smiling stewardess, and fell into a deep sleep. When he awakened and opened his eyes, he felt refreshed and full of beans. He was surprised to discover that he had slept for only about an hour, because he was convinced that it had been for longer. Upon raising the window blind, he noticed that the sun had not changed its position in the sky and was still on the left-hand side of the aircraft, at almost the same height as it had been when the plane left Tel Aviv. He spent the rest of the flight working, enjoying a light meal, and watching a movie, which sent him into another brief doze.

The landing at Kennedy International Airport in New York at noon local time was uneventful. His first business meeting was of some urgency and had been arranged for 6 P.M. local time the same day. When he reached the board room, he found that twenty people from all over the United States were waiting impatiently. As he made his presentation, he sensed that he was slowly losing his audience, his eyes closed occasionally, and he felt that sleep was overtaking him against his will. He glanced at his watch impatiently in the hope that the meeting would soon be over. Only then did he realize that his watch was still on Israel time and that it was 3 A.M.! Not only his watch was on Israel time: his body's clocks had also remained adjusted to Israel time. When the meeting had got under way, his body temperature had almost reached its lowest daily point and his sleepiness rhythm was at its height. For his body clocks, the seven-hour time jump that had been made during the eleven-hour flight from Tel Aviv to New York was too big.

The signs of jet lag became apparent not only in our businessman's falling asleep in the middle of the meeting, but also in the quality of his sleep that night. When the meeting finally ended at 9 P.M., our exhausted friend left for a night's sleep at his hotel. He fell asleep immediately but awoke at 4 A.M. Despite his overwhelming tiredness, he did not manage to go back to sleep and spent the rest of the night watching television. This early-morning awakening was also the fault of his body's clocks, which were still running on Israel time. He had awakened from his sleep at precisely the same time that he awakened at home on weekends after being up late the previous evening—about 11 A.M. The lack of coordination between his body's clocks and the environmental time markers had caused the disruption of his sleep and in his alertness and functional levels during the day. After a flight from Israel to the United States, most

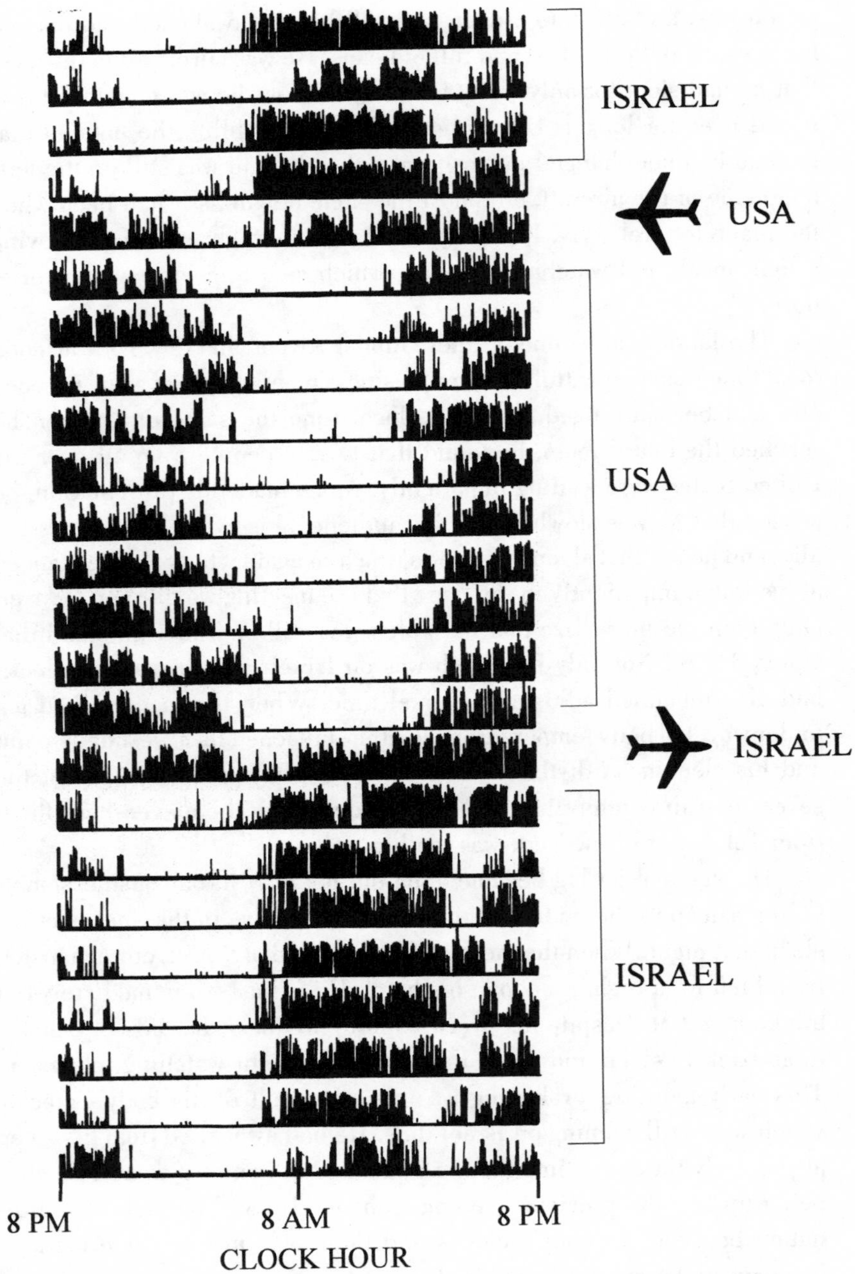
ISRAEL
USA
USA
ISRAEL
ISRAEL
8 PM
8 AM
8 PM
CLOCK HOUR

Fig. 33. Sleep-wakefulness cycle after a flight from Israel to the United States and back

people need three or four days to reestablish their coordination with the environmental clocks.

Although jet lag appears after flights in both directions—east to west and west to east—there is a great difference in the speed of adjustment between the two: it is slower after an eastward flight. As with the effects of the direction of the night shift workers' rota system on the workers' adjustment, the reason is to be found in the characteristics of the body's clocks. As we have seen, a person who goes to sleep at night according to New York time misses his sleeping time by seven hours, relative to the time he would have gone to sleep in Israel. If he goes to sleep relatively early—say, no later than 9 P.M. New York time—then his body clock will "show" 4 A.M. Israel time. At that hour it is very easy to fall asleep, and indeed, many people do just that after a late Saturday or Friday night party. The body clock of a traveler in the opposite direction who arrives on a direct New York–Tel Aviv flight and goes to sleep at his hotel at 9 P.M. Israel time is still on New York time and will "show" 2 P.M. Because of his fatigue after the long flight, he might possibly manage to fall asleep, but he will not sleep for long—two or three hours at most. This is because 2 P.M. is the time when the secondary sleep gate opens and sleep is very brief. If the eastward flight is at night and the passenger is able to sleep for a few hours, his first night's sleep in Israel will be even more problematic. A delay of sleep time from 9 P.M. to midnight in Tel Aviv will not improve the ability to fall asleep, for at midnight Israel time the hands of our American passenger's body clock are at 5 P.M. and, as we have already seen, it is most difficult to fall asleep at that hour. It is therefore recommended that aerial circumnavigation of the globe should always be from east to west!

It is almost certain that the wide variations in the adjustability of all kinds of people to jet lag stem from the interpersonal variations in the rigidity of their biological clocks, and from the effects of environmental time markers upon them. In the light of what is known about the rigidity of "early birds," it may be assumed that they suffer a great deal from jet lag, especially after eastward flights.

As we have seen, excessive sleepiness at times that we wish to be alert, difficulty in falling asleep, and difficulty in maintaining sleep continuity at the times we wish are the principal results of a lack of coordination between the body's clocks and those of the environment. One method of minimizing the effects of jet lag is planning sleep and wake-fulness times to take the lack of coordination between the two types of clock into account when flying either eastward or westward. On the west-bound flight, sleep time is delayed, so it is desirable to plan as follows: In the first few days after the flight west, it is preferable to advance bedtime to around 8–10 P.M. and then delay it gradually. I would therefore recommend that the traveler arriving in New York from Europe resist the temptations of the city's nightlife for the first few days, go to bed relatively early, and not succumb to the desire to sleep during the day.

There are two different approaches to the flight eastward. For the first few nights, the traveler can try to delay sleep time for as long as possible: if he goes to sleep at 5 A.M. in Tel Aviv, his body's clock will be at 10 P.M. New York time, a time at which he will be able to fall asleep—especially if he is tired and lacks sleep. This strategy is well suited to people who retire early. This way, they can advance their sleep time each day.

The second approach calls for splitting sleep into two periods during the first few days. The first sleep period can be adjusted to coincide with the opening of the secondary sleep gate at 3–4 P.M., or 10–11 P.M. local time. Although the sleep may possibly be brief, it will enable a delay of the second sleep period until the early hours of the morning local time. The two periods can then be gradually merged into a single sleep period.

In the future, it will be possible to utilize the effects of environmental lighting on biological clocks to enhance the treatment of jet lag. Travelers flying west will be exposed to bright light during the flight, causing a delay in sleep time. Those flying eastward will operate their "jet lag lamps" at specific times during the flight so that their body clocks will readjust to advance sleep time. Until commercial airlines equip their seats with high-intensity lamps, we suggest that travelers expose them-selves to bright sunlight for two or three hours immediately after landing. This natural source of light will ensure speedy adjustment to the condi-tions of the new environment.

# Children Who
# Refuse to Sleep

One of the tasks of sleep researchers who also happen to be parents is to lecture on sleep disorders at the various educational institutions attended by their own children. At the end of one such talk I gave to a group of parents at my daughter's kindergarten, I was asked, "What can be done with a child who adamantly refuses to go to bed and whose behavior at bedtime is simply impossible?" The agitated mother told me that her son was six years old and that the bedtime ritual began at 7 P.M. By 8 P.M., she said, "he has to be in bed." When I asked her, with raised eyebrow, why he had to be in bed at eight o'clock, she replied, "If he isn't, he disturbs our TV viewing." Despite my arguments, the mother found it difficult to understand why she could not get her son to bed at 8 P.M. and expect him to go to sleep against his will. When I asked whether she herself would be prepared to go to bed at 8 P.M., her indignant reply was, "But I'm an adult and he's only a child!"

Childhood sleep disorders are often the result of parental behavior and not of a sleep dysfunction in the child. Many parents impose sleeping habits on their children that are suited to the parents' life style but do not take the needs of the children into account. This usually stems from either a lack of knowledge or archaic beliefs and myths regarding sleep. Such parents are convinced that sleep is totally dependent on the will of the child, and so the fact that the child does not fall asleep at 7 or 8 P.M. is viewed as a lack of discipline or just plain mulishness. These parents cannot imagine that their child is unable to fall asleep so early because his sleep clock tells him to do so an hour or two later. By the same rule, there are parents who complain that their children wake up "too early," especially on weekends, thus disturbing their Sunday morning lie-in, and who find it difficult to accept the explanation that their child is not suffering from a sleep disorder but is simply reacting to going to bed too early. Children who go to bed at 8 P.M. will awaken at 5 or 6 A.M. because they do not need more than nine or ten hours of sleep. Therefore, one of the simplest ways of preventing childhood "sleep disorders" is to find the optimal sleep and waking-up time for each child. I am sorry to be the bearer of bad tidings, but sometimes the parents are called upon to sacrifice their own comfort in order to avoid friction with their children about sleep.

It should be added that not only parents are guilty of imposing sleep schedules that suit them more than their children; child-care specialists are guilty of it too. A few years ago the head of a residential home for children approached us for consultation concerning sleep disturbances in some of the children. Since these children were separated from their families for various reasons, she suspected that emotional reasons were behind their sleep problems. When we investigated their sleep, we were surprised to find that the main reason for the children's difficulties in falling asleep was the time they were put to bed: 8 o'clock in the evening. We recommended that the children's bedtime be delayed by one or one and a half hours, and the difficulties in falling asleep disappeared.

How, then, do we deal with sleep disorders of this kind at an age when it is still too early to tell the child to go to bed and sleep? As we saw in Chapter 5, the infant's sleep rhythm is consolidated during the first year of its life. Once the consolidation has been successfully completed, the infant sleeps during the night and remains awake during the day. But the rate of this process varies from infant to infant; some adjust rapidly and, much to their parents' joy, sleep at night when they are only a few months old, while others do not manage this even by the time they have reached two years of age. It is hard to believe how much emotion is bound up in the problem of the baby who refuses to sleep. I could fill another book with stories of exhausted parents who have tried every known technique to put their baby to sleep at night—from interminable rocking of the crib, through taking the baby for a drive around the neighborhood, to taking it out of the crib and cradling it in their arms. Every few weeks, these parents have to recharge their almost flat "sleep batteries" with a couple of nights at a hotel, far away from the screaming infant.

When analyzing such cases, we almost always find that the way the parents dealt with their rebellious infant helped determine the nature of the sleep disorder. Parents who had difficulty facing their baby's screams and tears did everything in their power to quieten him. As soon as he awakened and stood up in his crib, they stuck a bottle into his mouth, and if that did not work, they took him out of bed and cradled him in their arms or took him into their own bed until he fell asleep again. This was how the infant learned that all he had to do to gain his parents' attention was refuse to go to sleep, or wake up in the middle of the night and scream with the full force of his tiny lungs. Some parents made the courageous decision to let the baby cry until he calmed down, but the majority could not take the strain, surrendered quickly, and tried to pacify the infant by every means at their disposal.

The way to make the biological clock which controls sleep and wakefulness conform to the demands of the parents is by education and conditioning. Just as the ringing bell, which had no effect on the cat's sleep at first, gained special significance once it was combined with an electrical stimulus of the sleep center of the brain (see Chapter 13), so in children the entire gamut of stimuli and behavior that are part of the sleep ritual slowly become intimations of sleep. To assist this process, permanence and stability are of prime importance. A set bedtime should be maintained as part of an unchanging ritual that signifies the end of the day and the onset of night.

A baby whose place of sleep is changed from night to night—sometimes next to its parents, sometimes by their side on the couch as they watch television, and sometimes in their bed—will never "learn" the relationship between bed and sleep. The going-to-bed ritual is of cardinal importance at a later age too: the nightly customs which are maintained before the bedtime story or going to bed with various aids to sleep—a scrap of blanket, a piece of a broken doll, or a pacifier—are all part of a ritual that helps delineate the border between wakefulness and sleep, between day and night.

So what can be done about a baby who refuses to go to sleep? The way to deal with infants and toddlers who object to going to sleep is so simple that many parents do not even bother to try it because they are convinced that "it won't work."

From accumulated experience with babies in the Sleep Laboratory, we have found that there are two equally efficient methods at our disposal:

the "timed visit" and the "sleeping partner." Both methods were proposed by an English child psychiatrist named Naomi Richman. The first method calls for the infant to be placed in his crib with a few calming words and a cuddle or two; then, despite his protests, the parent leaves the bedroom. Ten minutes later, one of the parents goes into the bedroom, and if the baby is not in a comfortable position, he should be laid down, patted on his back, and left. This should be repeated precisely every ten minutes until the baby is asleep. This method should also be adopted if the baby awakens in the middle of the night. Avi Sadeh, who completed his doctoral dissertation on infants' sleep in my laboratory, examined the efficacy of this method by objective means. His experience has shown that an improvement, which is often dramatic, becomes evident in the babies' sleep after three or four nights. They fall asleep almost as soon as they are placed in their crib and begin to wake up less in the middle of the night; if they do awaken, they will not call their parents but will calm down by themselves.

With the "sleeping partner" method, one of the parents lies down to sleep on a couch or even on a mattress on the floor in the baby's bedroom, for a number of nights. A marked improvement in sleep behavior is shown after three or four nights with this method too, and the infant accepts the "sentence" of sleep without protest. It must be emphasized that both methods call for the parents to make a firm decision and then maintain the treatment unswervingly. This firmness has its rewards, for our records show that between 80 and 90 percent of the parents who have received counseling at the infants' clinic in our laboratory reported a marked improvement in their child's sleep during the first week of treatment. Many of them had raised a skeptical eyebrow when the method was first explained to them!

## AUTOMATISM IN SLEEP

Sooner or later, most children outgrow their sleep difficulties and conform to their parents' expectations. By age two, most sleep through the night, and sleep is continuous and restful through the rest of their childhood. Some aspects of children's sleep, however, are considerably less common in adults: sleepwalking, night terrors, bedwetting, sleep talking, and bed rocking. These sometimes strange automatic behaviors have puzzled physicians for centuries. But they have long been well aware of their characteristics, as is evident from Shakespeare's description of Lady Macbeth's sleepwalking:

> GENTLEWOMAN: Since his Majesty went into the field, I have seen her rise from her bed, throw her night-gown upon her, unlock her closet, take forth paper, fold it, write upon't, read it, afterwards seal it, and again return to bed; yet all this while in a most fast sleep.
>
> DOCTOR: A great perturbation in nature, to receive at once the benefit of sleep and do the effects of watching! In this slumb'ry agitation, besides her walking and other actual performances, what, at any time, have you heard her say?
>
> GENTLEWOMAN: That, sir, which I will not report after her.
>
> DOCTOR: You may to me, and 'tis most meet you should.
>
> GENTLEWOMAN: Neither to you nor any one, having no witness to confirm my speech.
>
> Enter Lady [Macbeth] with a taper.
>
> Lo you, here she comes! This is her very guise, and upon my life, fast asleep. Observe her, stand close.
>
> DOCTOR: How came she by that light?
>
> GENTLEWOMAN: Why, it stood by her. She has light by her continually, 'tis her command.
>
> DOCTOR: You see her eyes are open.
>
> GENTLEWOMAN: Ay, but their sense are shut.
>
> DOCTOR: What is it she does now? Look how she rubs her hands.
>
> GENTLEWOMAN: It is an accustom'd action with her, to seem thus washing her hands. I have known her continue in this a quarter of an hour. . . .
>
> DOCTOR: This disease is beyond my practice: yet I have

known those which have walk'd in their sleep who have died
holily in their beds.

*(Macbeth,* act 5, scene 1)

It would be difficult to find a more explicit description of somnambulism which underlines the extraordinary characteristics of this nocturnal behavior. Shakespeare engaged in some role reversal: it is the
gentlewoman, Lady Macbeth's servant, who enlightens the doctor about
the unusual features of sleepwalking and succeeds in touching upon each
of the most important symptoms of the phenomenon.

This sleep disorder, which appears mainly in adults under stress, is,
like all types of automatism in sleep, more common in children. It occurs
only during the deep sleep of stages 3 and 4. The sleeper suddenly sits
up in bed, gets down, and goes for a nocturnal stroll. The sleepwalker's
eyes are open wide but, as Shakespeare's gentlewoman indicated, they
are unseeing; he finds his way mainly by memory. If unexpected obstacles
are put in his way, he is likely to trip over them and fall. It is difficult
to awaken or communicate with the sleepwalker while he is sleepwalking.
Lady Macbeth's hand-washing movements are also not out of the ordinary
in sleepwalkers. During one of the rare somnambulistic events that occurred in the Sleep Laboratory, a charming little six-year-old boy sat up
in bed, got down from it as far as the recording electrodes that were
attached to him allowed, and began to wave his hands around with strange
and exotic movements. In the morning, when we watched the video with
his parents, we discovered that the reason for the hand movements was
far more prosaic: they were part of a school play in which the boy played
the role of the sun. There is, therefore, a tendency to reconstruct behavior
learned while awake during an automatic event that occurs during sleep.

Finally, the statement by Lady Macbeth's doctor that "I have known
those which have walk'd in their sleep who have died holily in their beds"
is correct. We do not view sleepwalking as a sleep disorder which holds
any risk or indicates an illness requiring treatment. The majority of children who walked in their sleep between the ages of five and thirteen
stopped gradually, and the disorder became part of family history. In
most cases, counseling parents how to deal with somnambulistic children,
together with an assurance that the sleepwalking will pass after a few
years, will suffice. As somnambulistic events occur during sleep stages

3 and 4, or the first two or three hours of sleep, parents can wait until the events actually occur and then help their children through them without any trouble. There is no cause to awaken them, for they will not respond in any case; all that has to be done is to direct them back to bed when they begin their walk. Most children will raise no opposition and will quickly fall back to sleep as though nothing had happened. In the morning, they will not remember a thing about their nocturnal adventures. A four-year-old girl from one of the kibbutzim in the Jezreel Valley, whom we saw in the Sleep Laboratory, used to "wake up" every night at 11 P.M., leave her bedroom, and walk to the kibbutz cowshed. In this case, sleepwalking held real physical danger, and practical measures to obviate the possibility of physical harm were called for. Another child, whose bedroom door led directly outdoors, would leave the house and cross a busy street. We recommended either that the bedroom door be locked or that the door handle be removed at night.

We do not usually conduct sleep recordings of somnambulistic children at the Technion Sleep Laboratory unless there is a possibility that the event is part of a nocturnal epileptic attack. One reason for this is that somnambulistic events rarely occur in a sleep laboratory. Sleeping in strange surroundings while hooked up to various electrodes seems to suppress automatic behavior. The majority of laboratory sleep recordings are conducted on youths on the eve of their conscription into the army. In cases like these, where there is a fear that sleepwalking might occur during military service, a complete probe must be undertaken before any medical or other steps are taken to deal with the sleep disorder.

Although "full-blown" sleepwalking is the most dramatic form of automatism during sleep, sitting up in bed and pulling at the covers— or just sitting up in bed with staring eyes—talking, making rhythmic movements, bedwetting (enuresis), teeth grinding (bruxism), and night terrors also fall into the category of what sleep researchers call parasomnias. The frequency of these nocturnal events may vary from once in a lifetime to several times a week. The factors common to all of them are their link to deep sleep, rapid transition from sleep to wakefulness, their tendency to pass at adolescence, and unconscious activation of motor mechanisms. Roger Broughton of Ottawa, who extensively studied automatism in sleep, termed them "disorders of arousal from sleep."

As we have seen, there is no call for therapeutic intervention in most

cases; parents simply need to be pacified and counseled about the significance of the disorder. This takes on a special meaning in the case of
night terrors. Parents who for the first time face a child who has awakened
from sleep because of a night terror experience an extremely frightening
event. They usually rush to the child's bedroom in response to blood-
curdling screams and find him sitting in bed with a glazed look on his
face, shivering. His raised pulse rate is clearly evident and it is difficult
to get the child to speak; he is detached from the environment and does
not respond. Even after he has awakened, he remembers nothing apart
from a vaguely threatening "animal" or "monster" that was "there in the
bushes" and attacked him. The erasure of the details of the night terror
from the child's memory is vastly different from the clear and detailed
memory of the nightmare, which originates in REM sleep. Here, too, the
only thing to do is to pacify the child and lay him down to sleep again.
There is no point in trying to get him to talk about it next morning and
thus heighten his fear that something is wrong with his sleep, because
he will not remember a thing in any case. Night terrors usually occur no
more than once or twice a month, and they gradually disappear in adolescence.

As Lady Macbeth's nocturnal wanderings illustrate, adults too can
suffer from automatism during their sleep. It usually occurs when the
subject is under stress and tension, and it tends to pass together with the
stress. In the event of frequent nocturnal events that do not pass, sleep
laboratory tests should be conducted to find the source of the disorder.

A form of automatic behavior in sleep which is unique to adults is
the REM behavior disorder described in Chapter 4. Patients who display
a plethora of violent forms of behavior, such as punching, kicking, or
rushing out of bed while enacting their dreams, may cause harm to themselves or to their bed partners. Medical attention should be sought in
order to avoid harmful consequences.


CLOSING THE LIFE CYCLE:
THE SLEEP-DISTURBED ELDERLY

Sleep disturbances at the two extremes of the life cycle—infancy and old
age—share the characteristic of being in many cases just another man-

ifestation of age-related changes. As a delay in the maturation of an infant's sleep-wakefulness cycle can be caused by parents' improper behavior, so an inappropriate response by elderly persons to the natural changes in their sleep may lead to severe sleep disturbances. The natural changes described in Chapter 4 render the elderly vulnerable to sleep disturbances. Therefore, they are more sensitive to what is going on around them while asleep: the twittering of birds, a car on the road, or even the light penetrating the slats of the window blind. But frequent awakenings from sleep are not caused by these stimuli, and the elderly continue to show increased awakenings from sleep even when they sleep in the complete silence of sleep laboratories or their own bedrooms. Therefore, complaints of sleep disorders at an advanced age do not necessarily point to a medical or mental disorder, but rather to a reduced quality of sleep brought about by the unavoidable process of aging.

"Sleep has changed for me," wrote Andy Rooney in a newspaper essay aptly entitled "Rock-a-Bye Baby Is Long Gone," and then went on to explain: "It's no longer a carefree, unconscious time for physical and mental resupply. I don't enjoy sleep the way I used to . . . maybe my memory is bad, but it seems as though I used to get into bed, go to sleep and wake-up eight hours later. If that was ever true, those days are gone forever. Now I go to sleep quickly but no longer sleep for long." Indeed, elderly people have great difficulty in maintaining consolidated sleep. They mostly suffer from fragmented sleep. Although one reason may be their greater sensitivity to what is going on around them, other explanations may be related to bodily changes that accompany aging. Interruptions of breathing during sleep and excessive leg movements in sleep appear in some 20–30 percent of elderly people. These changes, which may also indicate an age-related deterioration in the control over bodily functions, interfere with sleep, causing numerous brief awakenings. Likewise, waking up in order to urinate is very common in old age.

Recently, we found that the decrease in melatonin level, the "darkness hormone," which accompanies aging may also be responsible for sleep disturbances in the elderly. Iris Haimov, a doctoral student in my laboratory, investigated melatonin secretion in elderly people without sleep disturbances and in two groups of elderly insomniacs: those who lived independently and those who were institutionalized. She found that although there was no difference between the melatonin levels of healthy elderly and those of young adults, the insomniac elderly people had significantly lower levels of melatonin. This was particularly dramatic in the institutionalized insomniacs, who had hardly any detectable levels of melatonin. These observations led us to conclude that lower levels of circulating melatonin may be another cause of insomnia in the elderly. To test this hypothesis, we treated these melatonin-deficient elderly insomniacs with melatonin tablets. The results proved our hypothesis to be correct: treatment with melatonin shortened the time needed to fall asleep and enabled the elderly insomniacs to better maintain continuous sleep throughout the night.

There is no doubt that medical and mental illnesses can considerably exacerbate sleep disturbances in old age. This is particularly true in elderly people living in old-age and nursing homes. The absence of activities and interests in some of these places forces the elderly to retire to bed too early, which further aggravates their sleep difficulties. Since some of them are restricted in their mobility, they are not exposed to regular light-dark cycles. This may obliterate their melatonin cycles and further impair their sleep, as Haimov showed.

As an unavoidable consequence of their fragmented sleep at night, the elderly are increasingly prone to napping and dozing off during the day. It is very common to encounter elderly people napping on park benches, while riding a bus, or in physicians' waiting rooms. This multiple daytime napping, which compensates for some of the lost sleep at night, may further impair the elderly persons' ability to obtain proper amounts of nighttime sleep by reducing the sleep pressure.

In view of the above, it is not surprising that the rate of use of sleeping pills among the elderly is enormous, particularly in nursing home populations. Although misuse of sleeping pills exists among adults of all ages, the elderly patient is more likely to experience problems resulting from inappropriate use. First, there is an increased risk of toxicity in old age because of the body's decreased ability to metabolize and excrete the drug, and because of possible interactions with other medications. In fact, toxic drug reactions are one of the main causes of hospital admissions in old age. Second, because drugs remain in the bodies of elderly people for longer periods than in younger ones, they accumulate, bringing an increased risk of daytime side-effects. These may be in the form of agitation, loss of coordination, confusion, memory impairment, and even hallucinations. Because of the potentially grave consequences of sleeping pill misuse by the elderly, physicians must be certain that medication is really needed. In many cases, when sleeping pills are prescribed for an elderly patient, it is in fact the family or the nursing home staff who, annoyed by the patient's awakenings during the night, should be treated.

In sum, sleep is fragile at both ends of the life cycle. While in infants sleep episodes are yet to be consolidated into a single continuous episode that should also be adjusted to the environment, in old age the links between sleep stages are weakened and sleep is fragmented. Extra care should be taken to prevent the turning of these developmental changes in sleep structure into chronic and disturbing disorders.

# Excessive Sleepiness, or "In the Arms of Morpheus"

When we first began laboratory recordings at the Technion for the diagnosis of sleep disorders in the mid-1970s, I expected that the majority of the patients who came to the Sleep Laboratory for counseling would be suffering from insomnia or narcolepsy. To my surprise, it quickly became evident that most complained of chronic tiredness and a tendency to fall asleep during the day, especially in passive situations. Sometimes this tendency became almost unimaginably extreme. One of the first people to apply for counseling was the director of a large company. He complained of compulsive excess sleep and told us that when he felt himself falling asleep in the middle of long business meetings, he would take out his cigarette lighter and singe the soles of his feet under the table to prevent it. As proof of this, he showed me his blistered toes. To this day I shudder when I recall the complete equanimity with which he related this story.

The scientific literature in the mid-seventies that dealt with sleep disorders in the general population hardly touched on this type of complaint. In fact, researchers did not even ask about "too much sleep" or the tendency to fall asleep during the day. We therefore decided to study the incidence of excessive sleepiness and tendency to drowsiness in the population of Israel. But how can one conduct a reliable study of complaints which, on the face of it, are so trivial? It sometimes seems that statements like "I am very tired" or "I always want to go to sleep" are typical of the middle-aged Israeli male. Can we therefore determine that all males suffer from chronic excessive sleepiness?

In order to obtain reliable data that did not simply reflect

216

a state of mind but provided real evidence of a true disorder, we approached a large medical institute that conducted periodic medical check-ups on workers. Their tests included the completion of a detailed health questionnaire on the basis of which an interview with one of the institute's doctors was later held. Five of the one hundred questions that were posed dealt directly with sleep: (a) "Do you have difficulty in falling asleep?" (b) "Do you awaken frequently?" (c) "Do you use sleeping drugs?" (d) "Do you feel tired during the day?" and (e) "Do you sleep too much?" The subject was given four possible responses: (a) "never," (b) "infrequently," (c) "frequently," and (d) "always." As the subject knew that he would be extensively interviewed by the institute's doctor on the basis of his answers, it could be safely assumed that those who responded that they slept too much "frequently" or "always" really meant it and were not merely trying to make an impression.

When we analyzed the replies of all those tested by the institute in 1978—some fifteen thousand people in all—we discovered that four out of every one hundred people tested by the institute complained of sleeping too much. This percentage was much smaller than that of those who complained of difficulty in falling asleep and/or of frequent awakenings (18 percent), yet it was still much higher than any previously reported data in scientific literature. Unlike the complaints of "difficulties falling asleep" and "frequent awakenings," which were more prevalent in women than in men and whose incidence increased with age, complaints of too much sleep were more prevalent in men and were similar in all age groups.

These findings verified the impression we had received regarding the relatively large number of people who complained of excessive sleepiness and chronic tiredness and who did not usually gain the sympathetic ear they sought. It is easy to ignore complaints which appear to be banal. Many people told us about going to see the family doctor with a complaint of a tendency to fall asleep during the day, and being given a placatory or even dismissive reply such as "You're lucky that you sleep so well— I wish I could." Some told us that their doctor had recommended an extended vacation as a cure for accumulated tiredness, as if this were the only reason for their excessive sleepiness. Their claim that the tendency to fall asleep during the day only worsened on vacation did not usually gain any attention at all.

Once we had collated all the findings on the high prevalence of complaints about tiredness and excessive sleepiness, we had to try to determine the causes. One possibility was that the citizens of Israel did indeed sleep too little and therefore suffered from a chronic lack of sleep. In order to study this possibility in depth, we conducted a further study of fifteen hundred blue-collar workers. They were subjected to an extremely detailed interview that encompassed their sleeping habits, sleep disorders at night, disorders in their level of alertness during the day, the general state of their health, use of medication, job satisfaction, and more. The findings of our "industrial survey" on the incidence of complaints of insomnia, chronic tiredness, and excessive sleepiness corresponded almost exactly with the findings we had collected at the medical institute. Approximately 5 percent of the workers complained of an involuntary tendency to fall asleep during the day, especially in passive situations. But some cases were more serious. Some workers complained of a tendency to drop off during their breaks and worse, at work. We found significant connections between the complaints about the quality of sleep at night and the level of alertness during the day, and the entire gamut of factors related to work. Workers who complained about their sleep were less satisfied with their jobs, complained about a series of inconveniences at work—especially of tension in their relations with their coworkers—and pressure of work. But most important, a greater number of "sleepyheaded" workers were involved in work accidents than colleagues who had no complaints about their sleep.

To clarify the source of the complaints, we took a further step: we invited one hundred workers who had participated in the survey to undergo tests at the Sleep Laboratory. Happily, all accepted with alacrity. Our findings were unequivocal: the main reason for complaints of excessive drowsiness and tiredness during the day was respiratory disorders during sleep. Approximately half of the workers who had complained of excessive sleepiness and who were tested in the laboratory suffered from a respiratory disorder during sleep. When we compared these workers with their colleagues, we found a number of pronounced differences: respiratory disorders during sleep were definitely linked to hypertension, awakening with a headache, loud and bothersome snoring, and excessive body weight. We later found that all these factors are the most pronounced characteristics in people who suffer from sleep apnea syndrome.

A statistical analysis of the findings enabled us to determine with certainty that at least 1 percent of males over age twenty-one in Israel suffer from respiratory disorders during sleep. The estimate was much higher in the forty-to-sixty age group—approximately 3–5 percent. This was the first time that an estimate had been made of the population that suffers from respiratory disorders during sleep. Some years later, similar findings were reported in Italy, the United States, the Scandinavian countries, and Great Britain. These findings changed the face of sleep medicine completely.

## THE FIGHT FOR LIFE: THE SLEEP APNEA SYNDROME

My first encounter with a sleep apnea patient was when I was a postdoctoral fellow in Dan Kripke's sleep laboratory in San Diego, and it left a lasting impression on me. Strangely enough, the referral to the laboratory came in this case from the nursing staff of the internal medicine department to which he had been admitted. There were two reasons for the referral: first, according to the nurses, the patient was in a permanent state of sleep, while lying down, sitting, and even standing; and second, his extremely loud snoring kept the rest of the patients awake and had forced the nurses to put him in a room by himself.

Kripke agreed enthusiastically to examine the patient in the laboratory because his belief in the clinical possibilities of nocturnal recordings was not widely shared by the medical fraternity. The majority of his physician colleagues showed total indifference or dismissed the possibility that sleep could yield information that was more important than that obtained from a patient who was awake. The majority, and not only in San Diego, viewed what went on in sleep laboratories as just another kind of research that was conducted, by its very nature, at rather inconvenient hours.

The patient was extremely obese and had been hospitalized following complications resulting from hypertension. As medical literature contained evidence of obese patients who suffered from respiratory disorders during sleep, snored loudly, and tended to fall asleep during the day, we decided to conduct some special tests. Apart from the standard recordings of brain waves, muscle tonus, and eye movements, we tested the activity of the respiratory muscles and air flow in the nostrils. The results were amazing!

The moment the recording instruments showed that the patient had fallen asleep—that is, when the alpha waves denoting wakefulness were replaced by the theta waves of sleep stage 1—he stopped breathing for fifty seconds. Although it was clearly evident that he made a supreme effort to renew his breathing, something appeared to be stuck in his throat and blocking the passage of air. The patient was literally fighting for his life. He lifted his whole body from the bed in an effort to renew the flow of air. Suddenly, the "blockage" was freed and he began to breath again, emitting at the same time several prodigious snores, but a few seconds later he stopped breathing again. The brain wave recording showed that he had begun to breathe only after the brain waves indicating wakefulness had appeared; at the very moment he had fallen asleep again, he had stopped breathing. This cycle of apnea, a brief awakening, renewal of breathing, and another apnea recurred throughout the night; the patient suffered hundreds of apneas, each of which was terminated by a brief awakening and the emission of loud snores. In the morning, we counted more than 450 suspensions of breathing, each one having lasted for thirty to fifty seconds.

We asked the patient to return to the Sleep Laboratory next day in order to sleep during the day so that we could present this medical marvel to the hospital's staff. When we repeated the test, the doctors huddling around the recording instruments were unable to conceal their amazement at the drama unfolding before them in the adjoining bedroom. Some even expressed fear that the patient might die in his sleep, as though they were witnessing an isolated and extraordinary example of sleep, and suggested that we awaken him. It was difficult to convince them that the patient had slept this way for many years.

At the time, we had no idea of the sheer size of the revolution in sleep medicine these patients would cause. I do not know what became of our San Diego patient. Although his case caused great excitement and became the topic of conversation in the laboratory and the hospital cafeteria, it did not greatly change the laboratory's work. We continued to test the effects of sleeping drugs and study biological rhythms. That year we saw no more patients who suffered from sleep apnea syndrome. If

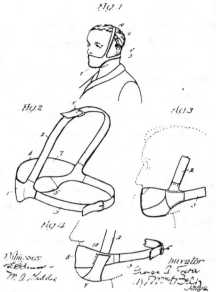

Fig. 34. A mouth harness to combat snoring, patented in 1917

anyone had told me that fifteen years later I would be seeing three or four new apnea patients every week, I would have laughed in his face.

When observing the sleep of an apnea sufferer, one is always troubled by the patients' obliviousness to their desperate nightly struggle. Only a few sleep apnea sufferers are aware of their condition. Their three main complaints—loud snoring throughout the night, morning tiredness, and a tendency to fall asleep during the day, especially in passive situations—may be explained by the nocturnal events they experience. The reason for the compulsive need to sleep during the day is the hundreds of nocturnal awakenings which interrupt their sleep. In order to renew their suspended breathing, patients are forced to awaken, sometimes for several seconds. A person who stops breathing some three to four hundred times a night awakens at least the same number of times and is therefore asleep for a total of no more than two or three hours. Over a period of years, this leads to severe chronic sleep deficiency, and it is hardly surprising that sleep apnea sufferers try to make up this shortfall during the day.

The loud snoring is also caused by respiratory disorders during sleep. The snorting sounds, which may be very loud and frightening, accompany the breaking of the obstruction in the airways when breathing is restored. The snoring is not continuous and monotonic but interrupted, with a "deathly silence" lasting for several seconds between one stentorian snore and the next. These silent periods, which appear to the apnea sufferer's bedfellow to last forever, are, in many cases, the direct cause of the decision to seek medical advice at the sleep laboratory. It is usually the woman who urges her husband to seek medical advice, whereas he, being totally unaware of the nightly drama, dismisses the possibility that he is suffering from an illness.

Additional complaints of sleep apnea sufferers are a dry mouth in the morning, mood and personality swings, lowered ability to concentrate, and a diminishing of intellectual powers. The majority of patients who have to struggle in order to renew their breathing do so with a wide-open mouth and renew their breathing through the mouth and nose at the same time. This is what causes the dryness and bad taste in the mouth. Unlike the nose, which is well equipped for the passage of air, the mouth is a relatively inefficient respiratory organ and tends to dry up. The changes in mood and behavior during the day can be ascribed to an extreme deficiency of sleep hours and a decrease in the supply of oxygen to the brain.

There are three main types of sleep apnea syndrome: central apneas, upper airway apneas, and mixed apneas. The central apnea is characterized by a disruption of the function of the respiratory brain center. The suspensions of breathing are suspensions not only of the airflow but of any respiratory effort. The respiratory brain center stops working for ten to forty seconds, thus causing a cessation of airflow. In the upper airway apnea, on the other hand, there is no absence of respiratory effort but only of airflow, due to a blockage in the area of the upper airways. In the mixed apnea, the suspensions of breathing begin as central apneas but conclude as an airway blockage. When airflow is stopped, the level of oxygen in the blood drops and the carbon dioxide level rises. These changes are registered by special sensors which are sensitive to blood gas levels and which transmit the information to the brain's control centers in order to renew breathing. In the upper airway apnea, this is manifested by an increasing effort on the part of the respiratory muscles to clear the blockage. The effort is evident in all the muscles of the patient's body; he sometimes raises himself on his elbows in a desperate struggle to renew the flow of air. It is therefore not surprising that he feels physically exhausted in the morning. In the much rarer central apnea, the renewal of breathing is accomplished without muscular effort and the lowered oxygen level in the blood is not as great.

While the airflow is being renewed, two more things take place: first, blood pressure becomes raised, sometimes radically, to extreme heights; second, variations, which are often dramatic, occur in the heart rate. During the apnea, heart rate is slowed considerably, but immediately after breathing is renewed, it accelerates sharply. In particularly severe cases, the apnea can cause a real heart dysfunction.

The drop in the oxygen level in the blood during the apnea is likely to affect the regular flow of oxygen to the brain and, as a result, its functioning. Evidence of this may be seen in behavioral changes and even diminished intellectual capacity.

Sleep apnea syndrome is prevalent in males, especially obese males. In our Sleep Laboratory, as in other laboratories throughout the world, the ratio of men to women among sleep apnea sufferers is ten to one. Although we have no convincing explanation of why women might be "immune" to sleep apnea syndrome, we can assume that two main factors are in play—hormonal and morphological. As the female sex hormone progesterone is a natural respiratory stimulant, it is probable that its secretion "protects" the woman against respiratory sleep disorders. The majority of women diagnosed as suffering from sleep apnea have passed menopause and no longer secrete progesterone. Some researchers also link this difference between the sexes with the structure of the upper airway, which is thicker in males. Whatever the explanation may be, it joins the wide range of differences in the incidence of disease between the sexes that have been reported in medical literature.


## THERE IS NOTHING NEW UNDER THE MOON

If sleep apnea syndrome is so prevalent and its characteristic symptoms so dramatic, then how is it that it was only discovered in the second half of the twentieth century? Were complaints of excessive sleepiness not discussed in medical literature before that? The first medical description of the syndrome was published in 1956 by Sidney Burwell, a renowned cardiovascular physiologist and dean of the Harvard Medical School, who reported on the relationship between respiratory difficulties during the day and compulsive falling asleep. The patient described by Burwell and his colleagues was so sleepy that he would fall asleep during card games—even when he held a great hand!—but Burwell did not ascribe his patient's falling asleep to a night sleep disorder. Only a few years later, when similar cases were examined in the sleep laboratory by French, German, and Italian researchers, did it become clear that all the subjects experienced numerous suspensions of breathing during sleep. This led to an accurate description of sleep apnea syndrome and a precise explanation of the reason for the extreme sleepiness which occurred during the day.

Yet a review of nineteenth-century medical literature shows that there is, so to speak, nothing new under the moon. Sleep apnea syndrome was described in some detail long before the sleep laboratory era, but for various reasons these descriptions did not attract the attention of doctors and therapists. Amazingly, when all kinds of physicians examined obese and drowsy patients, they almost always associated them with the same character—that of Joe, the boy servant in Dickens's *Pickwick Papers.* In the book, Mr. Pickwick is greatly impressed by fat, red-cheeked Joe's recurrent dozing off. Asked whether Joe sleeps all the time, he replies: "Sleep! . . . , he's always asleep. Goes on errands fast asleep, and snores as he waits at table. . . . I'm proud of that boy—wouldn't part with him on any account—he's a natural curiosity."

The character of Joe was doubtless in the mind of Richard Caton, who in 1889, at a meeting of the Clinical Society of London, presented the case of a thirty-seven-year-old poulterer who complained of great sleepiness which had appeared at almost the same time as a marked increase in his weight. "The moment he sat down in his chair sleep came on, and even when standing or walking he would sink into sleep," Caton wrote. "Constantly while serving customers in his shop, sleep would come on as he stood by the counter, he would wake and find himself holding in his hand the duck or chicken which he had been selling to a customer a quarter of an hour before, the customer having in the meantime departed." Caton's description of the poulterer's sleep leaves no doubt that he was suffering from sleep apnea syndrome:

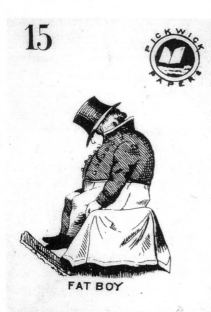

FAT BOY

Fig. 35. Dickens's "fat boy," Joe: from a popular English card game

When in sound sleep a very peculiar state of the glottis is observed, a spasmodic closure entirely suspending respiration. The thorax and abdomen are seen to heave from fruitless contractions of the inspiratory and expiratory muscles; their efforts increase in violence for about a minute or a minute and a half, the skin meantime becoming more and more cyanosed, until at last, when the condition to the onlooker is most alarming, the glottic obstruction yields, a series of long inspirations and expirations follows, and cyanosis disappears. This acute dyspnoeic attack does not awaken the patient. . . . If in the midst of the dyspnoeic attack he is forcibly aroused, the glottic spasm at once relaxes. The night nurses state that these attacks go on throughout the night.

Although the article in which this description was given was entitled "A Case of Narcolepsy," it was without doubt one of the first detailed descriptions of a patient who suffered from sleep apnea syndrome. At the conclusion of the discussion of the case, the society's president, Dr. Christopher Heath, pointed out the great similarity between the sleepy poulterer and Dickens's Joe. This similarity was noted by three other doctors, each completely unaware of the reports of his fellows. It is therefore no wonder that the combination of obesity and extreme daytime sleepiness has come to be known as the "Pickwickian syndrome." Today we know that Pickwickian syndrome is just one type of sleep apnea syndrome.

One of the earliest descriptions of the relationship between the type of breathing during sleep and a person's general health was given in the middle of the nineteenth century. It is found in *The Breath of Life* by George Catlin, an American artist and lawyer who tired of the legal profession and left his Philadelphia office to study the customs of the Plains Indians. One of his objectives was to learn the secret of the Indians' health. The Indians, said Catlin, were far healthier and stronger than the white inhabitants of the cities. According to Catlin, the only thing that separated the Indians' way of life from that of whites was the way they slept. While most Indians slept with their mouths closed and breathed only through their noses, many whites slept with their mouths agape because they breathed through their mouths while asleep. Breathing through the mouth while asleep, claimed Catlin, caused snoring, a feeling of tiredness in the morning, headaches, and increased susceptibility to illness. Breathing through the nose, on the other hand, gave a feeling of having had a good, refreshing sleep. The Indians would close the mouths of their children while they were asleep. God, Catlin wrote, had breathed "the breath of life" into the nostrils of man. Although *The Breath of Life*, illustrated with Catlin's amusing pictures, was published in five editions and won critical acclaim in contemporary medical literature, his contribution to sleep research was forgotten as the years passed by.

Others who described the relationship between regular breathing through the nose and quality of sleep failed to attract the attention of their contemporaries. One reason was the discovery of narcolepsy at the end of the nineteenth century. As a result, every person who had a tendency to fall asleep during the day was immediately diagnosed as narcoleptic. Such a decisive diagnosis, of course, left no room for further investigation. This is why as recently as the early 1980s sleep apnea syndrome—which affects some 3–5 percent of the male population between the ages of 40 and 60—was not even mentioned in medical school textbooks.

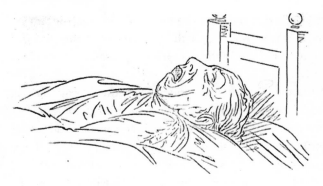

Fig. 36. Sleeping
with the mouth shut
and open: from
George Catlin's *The
Breath of Life*
(1861)

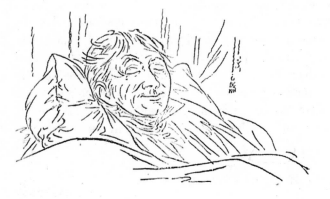

The conservatism of the medical profession offers another explanation for the ignoring of this phenomenon. In 1973, William Dement was unable to convince the doctors of a boy and girl suffering from extremely severe sleep apnea syndrome and resultant hypertension that he knew the reasons for their blood pressure problems and how to treat them. "Just like everyone else," said Dement, "doctors can be arrogant and pedantic." Only after the doctors had exhausted every possible treatment and the life of one of the youngsters was in real danger did they accept Dement's recommendation that a small puncture be made in the trachea. In those days, tracheostomy, which allows the blockage of the airway during sleep to be bypassed, was the most efficient treatment for sleep apnea. The results of the surgery were dramatic in both cases: the suspensions of breathing during sleep and the sleepiness during the day disappeared completely and the children's blood pressure returned to normal.

In Israel, too, the campaign to convince the medical profession of the high incidence of sleep apnea syndrome and its clinical significance was not easy. Many doctors saw no real significance in the findings of the Technion Sleep Laboratory. I shall never forget how, after a lecture on sleep apnea syndrome which I delivered at a national medical congress, a member of the audience rose and said: "My wife has counted two hundred apneas while I am asleep. Are you, who are not a physician, contending that I am ill?" He went on to lecture me, and the large audience of doctors, on the lack of significance of the number of apneas that occurred during sleep, claiming that he was a completely healthy specimen who suffered from neither sleepiness during the day nor sleeplessness during the night. He did not think that two hundred apneas a night were either a disorder or presented a danger of any kind. Yet that same doctor's physiognomy bore one of the telltale signs of the person who suffers from sleep apnea syndrome—a small, sunken chin and a very small lower jaw. Out of collegial respect, I elected not to reply.

## SLEEP APNEA SYNDROME: THE RISKS

On the face of it, the life of sleep apnea syndrome sufferers is in danger every night: failing to awaken from a single suspension of breathing would be enough to kill them by asphyxiation. But the brain's control mechanisms work so well that such a danger is extremely small. People who suffer from sleep apnea syndrome do not die of asphyxiation in their sleep unless they drink too much alcohol before bed or take large doses of sleeping drugs, both of which depress the activity of the respiratory brain center. But the health of these people is at risk for entirely different reasons. First, their tendency to fall asleep during the day leaves them wide open to accidents. One-third of those who have been diagnosed at the Technion Sleep Laboratory as suffering from sleep apnea syndrome told us that they had been in "near miss" situations as a result of diminished alertness while driving. Three percent admitted that they had been involved in car accidents because they had fallen asleep at the wheel. Studies conducted in various parts of the world have reported that more sleep apnea syndrome sufferers are involved in road accidents than those who do not have the syndrome. As the syndrome is so prevalent in males, there is no doubt that many professional drivers suffer from it. I am convinced that the day is not far off when periodic medical examinations of public-service vehicle drivers will include a test of the quality of their sleep, and especially their respiratory function during sleep, before the renewal of their licenses. Up to the time of writing, none of our efforts to spark the interest of the large public transport companies in Israel on this matter has met with success.

But falling asleep at the wheel is not the only danger facing sleep apnea syndrome sufferers. Their nightly struggles to renew their breathing have a significant effect on the function of their hearts and lungs. Nearly half of those who suffer from sleep apnea syndrome also suffer from hypertension, and there is much evidence that the syndrome is the direct cause of hypertension. These people are therefore exposed to all the illnesses and complications related to raised blood pressure. In a recent study, we found that the mortality rate of sleep apnea patients who died from heart attacks—22 percent—was nearly double that of the general population (13 percent).

Can we arrest the process by suitable treatment of the syndrome? We do not have enough data to provide a definite answer to this question, but it is clear that the younger the patient is, the greater are the chances of success. This is especially true of children suffering from sleep apnea syndrome which resulted from a mechanical blockage of the airway and resultant hypertension. The removal of the blockage caused an almost immediate return to normal blood pressure levels. Similarly, successful cures have been achieved in obese patients who lose a considerable amount of weight with the aid of surgery. With the disappearance of the apneas, a marked improvement in their blood pressure values and heart function is observed.

Although something of a revolution in doctors' attitudes to sleep apnea syndrome has occurred over the last ten years, I feel that the medical and public medicine establishments are still not dedicating enough effort and resources to combating the problem. Even by the most conservative estimates, we find that the United States has some twenty million sufferers from sleep apnea syndrome, the majority of whom are unaware of their condition. In the light of the syndrome's effects on day-to-day functioning and general health, the price paid by society is enormous.

The lack of awareness of the syndrome and its clinical significance is also apparent in the readiness to treat it. Many people who have been diagnosed in the sleep laboratory as suffering from the syndrome, and who have been referred back to their doctors for further investigation and treatment, call the laboratory complaining that the family doctor merely prescribed a sleeping drug "so that I would sleep better." A recent trace that we ran on the first fifteen hundred patients diagnosed at the Technion Sleep Laboratory between 1976 and 1988 showed that only 52 percent were given any kind of treatment for the syndrome. An examination of the change in the clinical condition of treated patients compared with untreated patients clearly showed that the condition of treated patients was far better. Yet recent years have revealed a heightened awareness of the subject both in Israel and abroad. The best evidence is that today in many countries medical students are required to demonstrate their knowledge of sleep apnea syndrome in their final examinations.

## SLEEP APNEA SYNDROME: METHODS OF TREATMENT

Since the seventies, when the first diagnoses were made, the treatment of sleep apnea syndrome has undergone many changes. As the most common form of the syndrome is the airway obstruction, the primary objective is to allow a normal flow of air during sleep. The first procedure to solve the problem completely was, as mentioned earlier, tracheostomy. A small puncture, which remained open during sleep and was closed during the day, was made in the windpipe. This circumvented the obstruction in the pharynx. Although tracheostomy was extremely efficient and solved the problem completely, the procedure was accompanied by side-effects and complications that limited its use to the most severe cases.

In less severe cases, surgical efforts were made to facilitate the passage of air by widening the airway. Doctors were inclined to believe that widening the airway would make counteracting the blockage easier. Thus, procedures for widening the nasal airways and removing enlarged tonsils, soft tissue, and even the uvula—the small, fleshy body that projects downward from the soft palate—are often used. Although these procedures did improve respiratory function during sleep to a certain extent, only a few patients were completely cured of the syndrome as a result.

Other treatments were based on weight reduction. Although it became clear that dietetic treatment was not usually effective, in cases of extreme obesity, massive weight reduction by means of surgery to reduce stomach size does cause the disappearance of the syndrome and the patient's complete cure. We examined more than seventy extremely obese sleep apnea syndrome patients at the Technion Sleep Laboratory. All of them underwent surgery, and after a drastic weight reduction—say, from four hundred to two hundred pounds—the apnea disappeared completely. But disappointment lay in store for us: seven or eight years after they had undergone surgery, we examined a group of these patients and found that half of them had put weight back on despite the surgery. Not only that, but the apneas during sleep had returned too.

The most efficacious treatment of sleep apnea syndrome was developed in the 1980s by a young Australian doctor named Colin Sullivan. His idea was so simple as to be pure genius: in order to break the blockage of the airway, he pumped air into the patient's nostrils through a mask worn over his nose. At the very moment that the air pressure reached a critical point, the apneas ceased as though by magic and the patient continued to sleep undisturbed. Happily, the Technion Sleep Laboratory was one of the first in the world to adopt Sullivan's technique, thanks to both the determination and the financial backing of one of our patients. Mr. H. was one of the first patients to be diagnosed in the Sleep Laboratory as suffering from severe sleep apnea syndrome. As his sleep recordings also showed a severe disorder of his heart rate, he underwent an immediate tracheostomy that resulted in the complete disappearance of the syndrome. But some years later, complications and infection made the closure of the stoma necessary, and this caused an immediate reappearance of the syndrome. Mr. H. then embarked upon a long series of surgical procedures which, in the end, did nothing to improve his condition. I mentioned the new Australian discovery to him, and without hesitation Mr. H. suggested that we try to contact Sullivan and examine the possibility of his coming to Israel with one of his new CPAP (continuous positive air pressure) machines. It goes without saying that Mr. H. offered to defray all the expenses involved. Fortunately, it turned out that

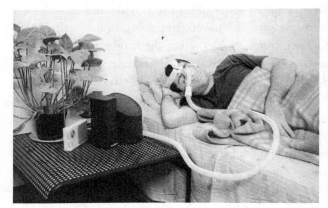

Fig. 37. A sleep ap-
nea patient sleeping
with a continuous
positive air pressure
(CPAP) machine

Sullivan's chief assistant, Dr. Ron Grunstein, had relatives in Tel Aviv.
Two weeks after our telephone conversation, Grunstein landed in Israel
with a large metal box containing the new wonder instrument.

As we quickly discovered, the most complicated aspect of preparing
the patient for respiratory treatment was the fitting of the mask. We had
to smear a thick layer of a rubber-like viscous compound over the patient's face, allow it to dry, and then peel it off and attach the air com-
pressor tube to it. Mr. H. was a tower of strength throughout this
procedure, and his reward was not long in coming. Once the patient had
fallen asleep, Grunstein gradually increased the air pressure inside the
mask to the point at which the apneas disappeared completely and the
sleep recording showed signs of turbulent REM sleep. But unlike the
first REM sleep of a normal night, Mr. H.'s REM sleep continued for
almost an hour and a half, which was longer than I had ever observed.
Grunstein was not surprised; he told us that one of the first observations
they had made of patients who had undergone this treatment was that at
the moment the apneas disappeared, an immediate entry into a prolonged
REM sleep or the deep sleep of stages 3 and 4 occurred. It is almost
certain that this is an immediate compensation for a long period during
which the normal amount of REM and deep sleep was prevented by the
apneas.

Upon awakening, Mr. H. spontaneously exclaimed, "That was a
dream of a sleep!" A few days later, Grunstein returned to Australia,

leaving the CPAP machine with Mr. H. A year or two later, the first machines for home treatment of the syndrome were developed. It was an American company which first saw the commercial possibilities of this treatment, and today thousands of CPAP machines produced by several different companies are sold every month. In Israel alone, more than two thousand sleep apnea syndrome patients are being treated by this method. Most of them use the machine nightly—it even accompanies them on trips abroad and while doing reserve service in the army. Neither they nor their sleeping partners can imagine what life would be like without the CPAP machine.

# Narcolepsy
## *Reversal of the Natural Order*

Excessive sleepiness during the day is not unique to sleep apnea syndrome; it is even more compulsive in the narcoleptic syndrome. Narcolepsy used to be the only sleep disorder about which one could read, albeit not a great deal, in medical literature. The reason for this is the dramatic character of the illness's symptoms. The narcoleptic patient suffers from uncontrollable attacks of falling asleep during the day. They can occur under almost any circumstances—while eating, during a telephone conversation, or while driving. The patient also suffers severe muscular laxity that causes collapse and falling. The combination of muscle laxity (called cataplexy) and attacks of sleep has in the past given rise to the suspicion that narcolepsy might be a form of epilepsy. This was the basis of the erroneous theory regarding the illness that found its way into several medical books.

Unlike the normal, healthy person or the person who suffers from excessive sleepiness as a result of a sleep apnea, especially under conditions of inactivity, narcoleptics suffer attacks of sleep when they are excited. A sleep attack may appear during an outburst of anger or joy, while laughing or crying, or even when the patient is surprised. The first narcoleptic to be examined at the Technion Sleep Laboratory said that the most annoying thing of all was that his attacks of "paralysis," as he defined them, always occurred when his grandchildren came to visit! Another patient, who was a teacher, told us that she never dared raise her voice to her pupils, as every loss of temper brought on an attack of muscle laxity and sleep. Much to her chagrin, her pupils exploited this to the full!

Two additional symptoms characterize some narcoleptics—hypnagogic hallucinations and sleep paralysis. Hypnagogic hallucinations, which are usually part of the falling-asleep process, appear in narcoleptics in the form of clear and detailed dreams which are often mixed with the last sights and sounds that the patient saw and heard before the attack. One of our patients suffered from uncontrollable sleep during bus journeys. She told us that the attacks were always accompanied by dreams in bright green; only years later did she realize that this was also the color of the seats on the bus. As I shall show, the dreams of narcoleptics can be fully explained by the character of their illness. In Chapter 3, I described sleep paralysis, which occurs when a person awakens with a feeling of acute paralysis that can last for a number of seconds or even minutes. This muscle paralysis, which characterizes REM sleep, overpowers the patient while he or she is awake and causes a deep sense of fear and helplessness. Many narcoleptics suffer from this.

Narcolepsy is not a new illness. Descriptions of narcoleptic patients can be found in nineteenth-century medical literature, and the phenomenon has even attained literary recognition. It is entirely possible that expressions like "my knees were knocking" or "he was paralyzed with terror" express the relationship between emotional excitement and paralysis. The first to put a name to the illness was the French physician Jean Baptiste Edouard Gelineau. On February 15, 1880, he saw in his clinic a Parisian wine-barrel merchant who complained of attacks of falling asleep at any time, as often as two hundred times a day! The attacks might take place during physical effort, when he was emotionally excited, and even when he was sexually aroused. According to Gelineau, the merchant, who had a healthy sense of humor, found it difficult to go to the theater, for every laugh would bring on an immediate attack. During his attacks of sleep, he experienced great muscular weakness, which on more than one occasion had caused him to fall in a manner reminiscent of a drunk or a child who falls asleep suddenly. Gelineau took great pains to point out that the collapse of the narcoleptic was caused by sleep, whereas in an epileptic attack sleep followed the patient's collapse. Despite the sharp distinction made by Gelineau, narcolepsy and epilepsy were confused for many years.

Since Gelineau first described narcolepsy, an overabundance of assumptions has accumulated regarding its source. At the beginning of the twentieth century, the illness was widely thought to be a mental reaction to pressure and frustration. Some viewed it as a defense mechanism against latent aggression, or even excessive sexuality: patients presumably escaped into sleep because they were unable to cope with their sex drives. This assumption was reinforced by the fact that the primary symptoms of narcolepsy appear in adolescence, when sexual and other changes occur. Narcoleptics were therefore given psychological treatment.

The first real breakthrough in the approach to narcolepsy occurred when the earliest sleep recordings were made of narcoleptic patients. Only then did it become clear that the structure of narcoleptics' sleep is vastly different from that of normal people. While the latter begin their sleep with sleep stages other than REM sleep, only reaching their first REM sleep after ninety minutes or so, the sleep rhythm of narcoleptics is reversed: they fall asleep directly into REM sleep. This reversal exists in both sleep at night and sleep during the day. When sleep recordings of attacks during the day were made, it was found that narcoleptics in fact suffer from attacks of REM sleep. This finding fully explained the strange characteristics of narcoleptic sleep attacks. It will be remembered that REM sleep is characterized by both muscle paralysis and dreams. In other words, the muscle laxity which attacks narcoleptics during an attack of sleep and the lucid dreams they report at the conclusion of their attack are part of normal REM sleep. But in contrast to normal, healthy people who remain unaware of events that occur during REM sleep, unless they awaken in the middle, narcoleptics who fall asleep directly into REM sleep during their daily routine cannot fail to be aware of them.

The fact that narcolepsy also exists in animals, especially dogs, has so far been of no help in solving the riddle. For some years now, William Dement has been raising a large group of narcoleptic dogs at Stanford University for purposes of research. At present, most of the evidence points to a disruption of activity in the brain stem, where the mechanisms which control REM sleep are located, as the main cause of the illness.

A further breakthrough recently caused excitement in scientific circles. For many years, evidence had come to light that if a family had one narcoleptic, the chances that other narcolepsy sufferers would be found in the same family were much greater than the chances in other families.

This had raised the possibility that the illness was genetically inherited. Then it was found that almost all narcoleptics have one thing in common: an exclusive genetic marker in their blood, the leukocyte antigen DR2 of the major histocompatibility complex. This marker, which is found in a small section of the general population, appears in the blood of ninety-nine out of every one hundred narcoleptics. This suggests that individuals who carry the genetic marker are predisposed to develop narcolepsy under as yet unknown conditions. Although genetic markers also characterize other illnesses, it appears that narcolepsy has the most specific one. This finding has diverted the study of narcolepsy to new and thrilling directions in recent years. Studies conducted in the last few years have shown that narcolepsy is probably not associated with a defect in a single gene. Based on the association of narcolepsy with the genetic markers in African-Americans and Caucasians, it has also become evident that the presence of DR2 in the blood, particularly in African-Americans, was neither sufficient nor necessary for the development of narcolepsy. Investigations of identical twins of whom only one suffered from narcolepsy also supported the idea that environmental factors which interact with the genetic factors play a critical role in the development of narcolepsy.

As far as I am concerned, the relationship between narcolepsy and genetic markers has solved one of the riddles regarding sleep disorders that has troubled me since the Technion Sleep Laboratory was opened. Based on experience acquired in sleep laboratories all over the world, I was convinced that the majority of people seeking counseling for excessive sleepiness would turn out to be narcoleptics. Although the exact prevalence of the illness in the general population is unknown, estimates suggest that there are three to four narcoleptics for every ten thousand people. In other words, we could expect to find at least fifteen hundred to two thousand narcoleptics in Israel. As the illness limits the functioning of the patient to such a great extent, it was also reasonable to assume that narcoleptics would be diagnosed at either their army induction physical or during their military service.

To my great surprise, the number of narcoleptics who came to the Sleep Laboratory was minimal—no more than twelve patients in twenty years! The possibility that the patients were being followed up by their own doctors and were therefore not in need of counseling at the Sleep Laboratory was rejected. In a survey which encompassed every neurologist in the country, we found that practically no new patients had joined the ones we already knew about. According to our findings, there are only twelve to fifteen narcoleptics in Israel—one hundred times fewer than we had expected. As there are big differences in the prevalence of certain diseases and illnesses among various ethnic groups, one possibility was that narcolepsy is not a "Jewish" illness. In order to examine the "Jewish question," I contacted a number of sleep researchers who worked in areas of the United States which had large Jewish populations and asked them, "Do you know of any Jewish narcoleptics?" Initially, they were somewhat insulted by the question: did I think that they explored the religious beliefs of their patients? Once I had placated them and explained why the information was so vital, I found that even at the Montefiore Hospital Sleep Laboratory in New York, which was for many years the only available sleep laboratory in the area containing the largest Jewish population in the United States, they had difficulty remembering a single case of narcolepsy in a Jewish patient. These findings were repeated in many other locations.

The relationship between the genetic marker and narcolepsy provided a partial solution to the riddle of why there are so few Jewish narcoleptics. It appears that there is a big difference between various ethnic groups regarding the prevalence of the genetic marker of narcolepsy. While in the United States and Europe some 20–22 percent of the population are carriers—in other words, the genetic marker is in their blood—only 9 percent of Israelis carry it. If it is assumed that narcolepsy appears because of an interaction between a genetic factor or factors and environmental factors, or some specific life events, then the number of potential patients in Israel is much smaller than in other parts of the world.

It is interesting to note that the highest incidence of the genetic marker in the world is in Japan. It is found in the blood of one out of every three Japanese, so it is hardly surprising that Japan has the highest number of narcoleptics in the world. Anyone who has visited Japan must have noticed the high level of sleepiness among the inhabitants. It is particularly noticeable while traveling on the subway: almost inevitably, half of the passengers are asleep in their seats. Although there is a tendency to ascribe the excessive sleepiness of the Japanese to their amazing industriousness, it is certainly possible that it is evidence of the influence of genetic factors. It is hardly surprising that the genetic marker in the blood of one hundred narcoleptics was first discovered by Japanese researchers Yutaka Honda and Takao Juji.

Narcolepsy is treated with stimulants that prevent the onset of the attacks of sleepiness. Use of these particular drugs must be under the supervision of a doctor. The attacks of muscle paralysis are treated with drugs which prevent the entry into REM sleep.


## THE SLEEPING BEAUTY SYNDROME

Greek mythology tells us the story of Endymion, a handsome young shepherd who fell asleep on the summit of Mount Latmos and was found by Selene, the moon goddess. She was unable to resist the charms of the handsome mortal and gave him her love. Zeus, the supreme deity of the Greeks, allowed Endymion to choose between two punishments: death or eternal sleep in which his youth would be preserved forever.

The folklore of many peoples is full of stories of heroes who fell asleep for months or even years. Nearly all of them awakened one day as though not even a single night had elapsed since they fell asleep. Rip van Winkle fell asleep and awakened after twenty years. Epimenides, a Cretan poet, fell asleep in a cave in his youth and awakened fifty years later to find himself the wisest man on the island. There are famous sleepers in every culture who awakened after their long sleep only when they were needed to fulfill a supreme national mission or to face their historic destiny. The British King Arthur awakened from his sleep on the enchanted isle of Avalon to face the Saxon invader. Ogier, the national hero of Denmark, and Frederick I, known as Barbarossa—who awakened from his sleep only when his beard had thrice encircled a large table upon which he had fallen asleep—are other notable sleepers. Don Sebastian, the Portuguese hero, also awakened to fight an invader—in this case, the Muslims.

Generations of children have gone to sleep while listening to the tale of Sleeping Beauty. She, and all those who dwelt in the palace, fell asleep for a hundred years after she had pricked her finger on the spindle. Only when the handsome prince kissed her on the cheek did all the sleepers awaken and live happily ever after. The story of Sleeping Beauty, which

was first published in the seventeenth century in a book written by
Charles Perrault, reappeared almost a century later, in nearly identical
form, in the Grimm brothers' fairy tales.

Is there any factual foundation to the myths and folktales of sleeping
heroes? Medical literature of the last century contains descriptions of
famous sleepers who slept for months and even years and who could not
be awakened. It is interesting to note that most of them were young girls
who attained both fame and nicknames, like "The Girl of Montrose" or
"Sleeping Effie." Some observers noted the similarity between the sleeping girls and those who starved themselves to death, an illness that is
well known today as anorexia nervosa and which was first described in
1872. Others likened prolonged sleep in humans to the hibernation of
bears in the northern regions.

The only scientific documentation of awakening from a prolonged
sleep, something like that of Sleeping Beauty, was made of patients suffering from the "sleeping sickness" discovered by von Economo, encephalitis lethargica, which I described in Chapter 13. Oliver Sacks, in
his book *Awakenings*, documented the effects of treatment with L-dopa
on patients suffering from "sleeping sickness." For many years these
patients "lay motionless and without speaking, and in some cases were
almost devoid of desire and thought . . . it was as though their entire being
was enveloped or sealed into a bubble." Sacks goes on to describe the
awakening of one of the patients: "After twenty years of motionlessness
and introversion, she burst out and landed in the air like a cork that had
been released from the depths. . . . [When this happened] I thought of a
spring awakening after the winter sleeps; I thought of Sleeping Beauty."
Although we have no conclusive proof, it is probable that some of the
cases of prolonged sleep described in medical literature one and two
hundred years ago were of isolated cases of encephalitis lethargica or
similar illnesses. The sleepers got well spontaneously. It is also probable
that cases like this were the inspiration behind the folk stories.

Although we have not seen even a single case of the Sleeping Beauty
syndrome in the Technion Sleep Laboratory, we have encountered cases
characterized by episodes of prolonged sleepiness, or the Kleine-Levin
syndrome. This syndrome was first identified some sixty years ago by two
psychiatrists, Willi Kleine in Germany and Max Levin in New York, who
described youths suffering from prolonged sleepiness and extreme over-

eating. These and cases reported later had common characteristics: nearly all the patients were young males between the ages of fifteen and twenty-five who, apart from the attacks of sleepiness, suffered from severe behavioral disturbances.

At the Sleep Laboratory we have seen some twenty people suffering from the syndrome—far more than those found in any other sleep laboratory in the world. Although there was a great similarity in the patients' stories regarding the attacks of sleepiness, we found large variations in the way the syndrome appeared from patient to patient. With some patients, the attacks of sleepiness appeared with extreme precision each week, for two or three days at a time, while in others the attacks appeared only three or four times a year, for a week at a time. In the majority of the patients, the behavioral disturbances that accompanied the attacks of sleepiness were related to compulsive eating and aberrant sexual behavior. In some cases, the behavioral deviations were surprising in their strangeness. I recall a conversation with the mother of a fourteen-year-old boy who had been referred to the Sleep Laboratory because every few months he would fall into a sleep for three or four days from which it was impossible to awaken him. The mother asked to talk to me in private about additional symptoms that had caused her to think that her son had lost his mind. According to her, the first signs of an impending attack of sleepiness were changes in her son's behavior. The likable and well-behaved youngster, "who had never been given a bad mark for conduct at school," would suddenly become an unknown stranger. He would undress and walk around the house naked, especially when his mother's friends came to call. She found him masturbating, with no attempt at concealment, in various rooms in the house. He was afraid of venturing out of the house because "there are enemies waiting to kill me outside." Immediately before the onset of the attack of sleepiness, he would go to the refrigerator and ravenously devour its contents. I think that any mother would be filled with horror under such circumstances. One of the most surprising things that recurred throughout all the patients' stories was the suddenness with which the attack appeared and subsided. At the onset of the attack, it seemed that an invisible hand had turned off a switch in the boy's brain, and in a split second he had turned from Dr. Jekyll into Mr. Hyde. After a few days, the switch was turned on, Mr. Hyde disappeared and Dr. Jekyll took his place once more.

We have no explanation of the source of the Kleine-Levin syndrome, but the thread leads us to that same minuscule location in the brain called the hypothalamus. It is the hypothalamus that controls our drives, the activity of the autonomic nervous system and sleep. It is so small that it cannot be reached directly in order to study it. One of the indirect ways in which we can learn about how it functions is through the hormonal system. As the hypothalamus also controls the secretion of various hormones, any disruption in these secretions may teach us about a possible dysfunction of the hypothalamus. In a joint study with some colleagues from the Beilinson Hospital in Petach-Tikva, Israel, we found disruptions in the secretions of prolactin and the gonadotropines—which are under the control of the hypothalamus—in a twenty-three-year-old Kleine-Levin syndrome patient. This indicates a general disruption of hypothalamic control, which affects sleep and causes behavioral disturbances that are related to drives like hunger, thirst, and sex. It would appear that the disruption is related to the removal of the inhibitors of the activity of the various centers in the hypothalamus. When the inhibitors are no longer in place, the patient tries to satisfy his drives without thought to societal or moral norms.

Although we are able to describe the syndrome with such precision and even postulate its source, we still do not understand why it occurs in cyclic form, and as yet we have no efficient treatment for its prevention. Various stimulants have been tried unsuccessfully. In most cases, there is nothing to do apart from trying to pacify the horror-stricken parents by assuring them that once the attack has passed, their son will return to normal. And yet there is some small comfort in the knowledge that whereas the severity of narcolepsy remains unchanged throughout the life of the patient, there is an ever-increasing improvement in cases of Kleine-Levin syndrome. The frequency of the attacks diminishes, their duration is shortened, and they often disappear completely after several years.

In summary, excessive daytime sleepiness is no laughing matter. It may appear in different forms, ranging from a tendency to snooze in boring, passive situations to the abrupt and embarrassing sleep spells of the narcoleptic and the prolonged sleeping periods of the Kleine-Levin patient. In all these cases, the delicate balance between sleep and wakefulness has been disrupted, and in order to treat it the source of the excessive sleepiness must be correctly diagnosed.

# Epilogue

Looking back, sleep researchers can allow themselves to feel a great deal of satisfaction. There are very few fields of research in which so much progress has been made in such a short space of time. Although we still do not have conclusive answers to the question of why we sleep and dream, the scraps of information that have been gleaned during thousands of nights spent in sleep laboratories have started to crystallize.

But what does the future hold, and what will sleep research reveal in the twenty-first century? Since the 1960s the number of sleep researchers has steadily increased, but it would appear that the golden era of earth-shaking discoveries has passed. Then, every night held the chance of a new and thrilling revelation, with researchers anxiously awaiting the morning so that they could report on the night's findings.

Today there is a more sober attitude toward our ability to explain events occurring in the sleeping brain, whether it be through a neurotransmitter or in a single nerve center. Michel Jouvet described this sobering up beautifully at the inaugural congress of the International Organization for Sleep Research in 1991. He told us then that he regarded the neurotransmitter serotonin, which in the sixties he had viewed as being responsible for sleep, as a "second-rate novel." At first, he said, it was a torrid love affair. Every experiment he conducted was crowned with success and he was convinced that it was the secretion of serotonin that facilitated the transition from wakefulness to sleep. Then came the years of doubt and suspicion. Further experimenting proved that serotonin, and the nerve cells in the brain which contained it, failed to conform to his theory. It was found that the nerve cells were active during wakefulness and that the release of serotonin from them did not occur during sleep. Jouvet then decided to abandon his research on the relationship between serotonin and sleep, directing his efforts to other fields. Only recently did he return to his original idea. Today, Jouvet is again convinced that serotonin is indeed related to sleep, but in a far more complex and complicated way than he first imagined.

The last decade of the twentieth century was designated by President George Bush, amid much ceremony, as the Decade of the Brain. This declaration was a political recognition of something that scientists had known for many years—that the human brain is the most complicated, complex, and wonderful creation in the entire universe. In this context, I am convinced that research on the alert brain cannot be separated from that on the sleeping brain. Future understanding of the functioning of the sleeping brain will undoubtedly progress in parallel with understanding of the functioning of the alert or wakeful brain. However, in contrast to the slow progress in understanding the remarkable brain mechanism that leads to sleep and dreams, recognition of the importance of sleep medicine is slowly but surely trickling down to every field of medicine.

Within a few years, I believe that nights spent in the sleep laboratory will become a matter of routine, just like any other medical tests. The day will come when workers who need a specially high level of alertness and preparedness (nuclear reactor operators, air traffic controllers, pilots, and public-service vehicle drivers, for example), and who show signs of excessive sleepiness and fatigue, will have to undergo periodic sleep tests to show whether they have a sleep disorder which might impair their efficient functioning.

Treatment of sleep disorders will also undergo great changes. No longer will sleeping drugs automatically be prescribed for people who complain of insomnia; instead, a precise examination will become standard practice before any treatment is undertaken. Laboratory discoveries of a wide range of natural compounds in the brain, and related to sleep, will be the start of the development of new, natural sleeping preparations.

It is possible that in the next century we will be able to buy home instruments which will trace the activity of our sleep rhythms, and biological alarm clocks which will enable us to wake up at any stage of sleep. Maybe setting a biological alarm clock to REM sleep will enable those who are interested to compile entire "libraries" of dreams.

And what of the possibility that in the future we will be able to shorten our sleep drastically—or even exist without it? I'm sorry to disappoint you, but I cannot believe that a world without sleep is possible.

It was not without good reason that my mentor, Bernie Webb, called sleep the "gentle tyrant." It will continue, so it seems, to dominate us, softly and ethereally, until the end of time.

# References

General

      Anch, A. M., et al. 1988. *Sleep: A scientific perspective.* Englewood Cliffs, N.J.: Prentice-Hall.

      Borbely, A. *Secrets of sleep.* 1986. New York: Basic.

      Carskadon, M. A., ed. 1993. *Encyclopedia of sleep and dreaming.* New York: Macmillan.

      Dement, W. C. 1976. *Some must watch while some must sleep.* San Francisco: San Francisco Book Company.

      ————. 1992. *The sleepwatchers.* Stanford, Calif.: Stanford Alumni Association.

      Hobson, J. A. 1989. *Sleep.* New York: Scientific American Library.

      Horne, J. 1988. *Why we sleep.* New York: Oxford University Press.

      Kleitman, N. 1963. *Sleep and wakefulness.* Chicago: University of Chicago Press.

      Webb, W. B. 1975. *Sleep: The gentle tyrant.* Englewood Cliffs, N.J.: Prentice-Hall.

Chapter 1. Sleep and Death

      Aristotle. 1964. *On sleeping and waking.* Trans. W. S. Hett. Cambridge: Harvard University Press.

      Lucretius. 1959. *On the nature of the universe.* Trans. R. E. Latham. Baltimore: Penguin.

      Morruzi, G. 1962. The historical development of the deafferentation hypothesis of sleep. *Proceedings of the American Philosophical Society* 108:19–28.

      Renshaw, S., U. L. Miller, and D. P. Marquis. 1933. *Children's sleep.* New York: Macmillan.

      Schiller, F. 1982. Semantics of sleep. *Bulletin of the History of Medicine* 6:377–97.

      Wittern, R. 1989. Sleep theories in antiquity and the Renaissance. In J. A. Horne, ed. *Sleep '88,* pp. 11–22. Stuttgart: Fischer.

Chapter 2. Brain Waves

Brazier, M. A. B. 1961. *A history of the electrical activity of the brain: The first half-century.* London: Pitman.

————. 1984. *A history of neurophysiology in the seventeenth and eighteenth centuries.* New York: Raven.

Carskadon, M. A., and W. C. Dement. 1989. Normal human sleep: An overview. In M. H. Kryger, T. Roth, and W. C. Dement, eds. *Principles and practice of sleep medicine,* pp. 3–13. Philadelphia: Saunders.

Davis, H., et al. 1938. Human brain potentials during the onset of sleep. *Journal of Neurophysiology* 1:24–38.

Johnson, L. C. 1973. Are stages of sleep related to waking behavior? *American Scientist* 61:326–38.

Ogilvie, R. D., and R. T. Wilkinson. 1984. The detection of sleep onset: Behavioral and physiological convergence. *Psychophysiology* 21:510–20.

Rechtschaffen, A., and A. Kales. 1968. *Manual of standardized terminology, techniques and scoring system for sleep stages of human subjects.* National Institutes of Health Publications no. 204. Washington, D.C.: NIH.

Webb, W. B., and H. W. Agnew, Jr. 1971. Stage 4 sleep: Influence of time course variables. *Science* 174:1354–56.


Chapter 3. Nathaniel Kleitman

Aserinsky, E., and N. Kleitman. 1953. Regularly occurring periods of eye motility, and concomitant phenomena during sleep. *Science* 118:273–74.

Dahlitz, M., and J. D. Parkes. 1993. Sleep paralysis. *Lancet* 341:406–7.

Fisher, C., J. Gross, and J. Zuch. 1965. Cycle of penile erection synchronous with dreaming (REM) sleep. *Archives of General Psychiatry* 12:29–45.

Jouvet, M., and M. Michel. 1959. Correlation electromyographiques du sommeil chez le chat décortique et mesencephalique chronique. *Comptes rendus des séances de la Société de Biologie et de ses filiales* (Paris) 153:422–25.

Snyder, F., et al. 1964. Changes in respiration, heart rate, and systolic blood pressure in human sleep. *Journal of Applied Psychology* 19:417–22.

Vogel, G. An interview with Nathaniel Kleitman. Archival Video Histories of Sleep Researchers. Available from Brain Information Service, UCLA School of Medicine, Los Angeles, Calif., 90024–1761.


Chapter 4. The Rhythm of Sleep

Boyar, R., et al. 1972. Synchronization of augmented luteinizing hormone secretion with sleep during puberty. *New England Journal of Medicine* 287: 582–86.

Coons, S., and C. Guilleminault. 1982. Development of sleep-wake patterns and non-rapid eye movement sleep stages during the first six months of life in normal infants. *Pediatrics* 69:793–98.

Granat, M., et al. 1979. Short-term cycles in human fetal activity. Part 1: Normal pregnancies. *American Journal of Obstetrics and Gynecology* 134:696–701.

Knobil, E., et al. 1980. Neuroendocrine control of the rhesus monkey menstrual cycle: Permissive role of the hypothalamic gonadotropin releasing hormone (GnRH). *Science* 207:1371–73.

Sterman, M. B., and T. Hoppenbrouwers. 1971. Development of sleep-waking and rest-activity patterns from fetus to adult in man. In M. B. Sterman, D. J. McGinty, and A. Adinolfi, eds. *Brain development and behavior.* New York: Academic Press.

Takahashi, Y., D. M. Kipnis, and W. H. Daughaday. 1968. Growth hormone secretion during sleep. *Journal of Clinical Investigation* 47:2079–90.

Webb, W. B. 1982. Sleep in older persons: Sleep structure of 50- to 60-year-old men and women. *Journal of Gerontology* 37:581–86.

Weitzman, E. D., et al. 1971. Twenty-four-hour pattern of the episodic secretion of cortisol in normal subjects. *Journal of Clinical Endocrinology* 33:14–22.

Williams, R. L., H. W. Agnew, Jr., and W. B. Webb. 1964. Sleep patterns in young adults: An EEG study. *Electroencephalography and Clinical Neurophysiology* 17:376–81.

Chapter 5. The Twenty-five Hour Day

Aschoff, J. 1965. Circadian rhythms in man. *Science* 148:1427–32.

Aschoff, J., and R. Wever. 1976. Human circadian rhythms: A multioscillatory system. *Federation Proceedings* 35: 2326–32.

Czeisler, C. A., et al. 1980. Human sleep: Its duration and organization depend on its circadian phase. *Science* 210:1264–1267.

Daan, S., S. G. D. Beersma, and A. A. Borbely. 1984. Timing of human sleep: Recovery process gated by a circadian pacemaker. *American Journal of Physiology* 246:R161–78.

Dinges, D. F., and R. J. Broughton, eds. 1989. *Sleep and alertness: Chronobiological, behavioral and medical aspects of napping.* New York: Raven.

Lavie, P. 1986. Ultrashort sleep-waking schedule. Part 3: "Gates" and "forbidden zones" for sleep. *Electroencephalography and Clinical Neurophysiology* 63:414–25.

Lavie, P., and W. B. Webb. 1975. Time estimates in a long-term time-free environment. *American Journal of Psychology* 88:177–86.

Lavie, P., and A. Zvuluni. 1992. The 24-hour sleep propensity function: Experimental bases for somnotypology. *Psychophysiology* 29:566–75.

Richardson, G. S., et al. 1982. Circadian variation of sleep tendency in elderly and young adult subjects. *Sleep* 5:S822-S894.

Siffre, M. 1965. *Beyond time.* London: Chatto and Windus.

———. 1975. Six months alone in a cave. *National Geographic* 147:426–35.

Wever, R. A. 1979. *The circadian system of man.* Berlin: Springer.

Wollman, M., and P. Lavie. 1986. Hypernychthemeral sleep-wake cycle: Some hidden regularities. *Sleep* 9:324–34.

Chapter 6. From Sun Clocks to Biological Clocks

Altschule, M. D., and I. J. Kitay. 1954. *The pineal gland: A review of the physiological literature.* Cambridge: Harvard University Press.

Arendt, J. 1988. Melatonin. *Clinical Endocrinology* 29:205–29.

Czeisler, C. A., and C. Guilleminault. 1979. 250 years ago: Tribute to new discipline (1729–1979). *Sleep* 2:155–60.

Czeisler, C. A., et al. 1986. Bright light resets the human circadian pacemaker independent of the timing of the sleep wake cycle. *Science* 233:667–71.

Hippocrates. 1989. *The genuine works of Hippocrates.* Trans. F. Adams. Baltimore: Williams and Wilkins.

Lavie, P. 1992. Two 19th-century chronobiologists: Thomas Laycock and Edward Smith. *Chronobiology International* 9:83–96.

Lerner, A. B., et al. 1958. Isolation of melatonin, the pineal gland factor that lightens melanocytes. *Journal of the American Chemical Society* 80:2587.

Lewy, A. J., et al. 1980. Light suppresses melatonin secretion in humans. *Science* 210:1267–69.

Miles, L., et al. 1977. Blind man living in normal society has circadian rhythms of 24.9 hours. *Science* 198:421–23.

Moore-Ede, M. C., C. A. Czeisler, and G. S. Richardson. 1983. Circadian timekeeping in health and disease. Part 1: Basic properties of circadian pacemakers. *New England Journal of Medicine* 309:469–76.

Moore-Ede, M. C., F. M. Sulzman, and C. A. Fuller. 1982. *The clocks that time us.* Cambridge: Harvard University Press.

Richter, C. P. *Biological clocks.* 1965. Springfield, Ill.: Charles C. Thomas.

Tzischinsky, O., A. Shlitner, and P. Lavie. 1993. The association between the nocturnal sleep gate and nocturnal onset of urinary 6-sulfatoxymelatonin. *Journal of Biological Rhythms* 8:199–209.

Tzischinsky, O., et al. 1991. Circadian rhythms in 6-sulfatoxymelatonin and nocturnal sleep in blind children. *Chronobiology International* 8:168–75.

Winfree, A. T. 1987. *The timing of biological clocks.* New York: Scientific American Library.

Chapter 7. Dreams: Creatures of the Brain

Dement, W., and N. Kleitman. 1957. The relation of eye movements during sleep to dream activity: An objective method for the study of dreaming. *Journal of Experimental Psychology* 53:339–46.

Domhoff, B., and J. Kamiya. 1964. Problems in dream content study with objective indicators. Part 3: Changes in dream content throughout the night. *Archives of General Psychiatry* 11:529–35.

Foulkes, D. 1962. Dream reports from different stages of sleep. *Journal of Abnormal and Social Psychology* 65:14–25.

Freud, S. 1953. *The interpretation of dreams* (1900). Vol. 4, part 5 of J. Strachey, trans. and ed. *The standard edition of the complete psychological works of Sigmund Freud.* London: Hogarth.

Hall, C. S., et al. 1982. The dreams of college men and women in 1950 and 1980: A comparison of dream contents and sex differences. *Sleep* 5:188–194.

Hall, C. S., and R. Van de Castle. 1966. *The content analysis of dreams.* New York: Appleton, Century, Crofts.

Hobson, J. A., and R. W. McCarley. 1977. The brain as a dream state generator: An activation-synthesis hypothesis of the dream process. *American Journal of Psychiatry* 134:1335–48.

Jouvet, M. 1979. Mémoires et "cerveau dédoublé" au cours du rêve. *Revue du praticien* 29:27–32.

———. 1992. *Le sommeil et le rêve.* Paris: Odile Jacob.

Lavie, P., and J. A. Hobson. 1986. The origin of dreams. *Psychological Bulletin* 100:229–240.

Lincoln, J. S. 1935. *The dream in primitive cultures.* London: Cressett.

Mack, E. M. 1974. *Nightmare and human conflict.* Boston: Houghton Mifflin.

Nielsen, T. A., and R. A. Powell. 1989. The "dream-lag" effect: A 6-day temporal delay in dream content incorporation. *Psychiatric Journal of the University of Ottawa* 14:561–65.

Offenkrantz, W., and A. Rechtschaffen. 1963. Clinical studies of sequential dreams. Part 1: A patient in psychotherapy. *Archives of General Psychiatry* 8:497–508.

Snyder, F. 1963. The new biology of dreaming. *Archives of General Psychiatry* 8:381–91.

Van de Castle, R. L. 1971. *The psychology of dreaming.* Morristown, N.J.: General Learning Press.

Chapter 8. Alfred Maury and the Dream of the Guillotine

Berger, R. J., P. Olley, and I. Oswald. 1962. The EEG, eye movements and dreams of the blind. *Quarterly Journal of Experimental Psychology* 14:183–86.

Berger, R. J., and I. Oswald. 1962. Eye movements during active and passive dreams. *Science* 137:601.

Dagan, Y., P. Lavie, and A. Bleich. 1991. Elevated awakening thresholds in sleep stage 3–4 in war-related post-traumatic stress disorder. *Biological Psychiatry* 30:618–22.

Dement, W. C., and E. A. Wolpert. 1958. The relation of eye movements, body motility and external stimuli to dream content. *Journal of Experimental Psychology* 55:543–53.

Foulkes, D. 1967. Nonrapid eye movement mentation. *Experimental Neurology* suppl. 4:28–38.

Goodenough, D. 1991. Dream recall: History and current status of the field. In S. Ellman and J. S. Antrobus, eds. *The mind in sleep.* 2d ed., pp. 143–71. New York: Wiley Interscience.

Gross, M., and P. Lavie. 1994. Dreams in sleep apnea patients. *Dreaming* 4:195–204.

Hefez, A., L. Metz, and P. Lavie. 1987. Long-term effects of extreme situational stress on sleep and dreaming. *American Journal of Psychiatry* 144:344–47.

Herman, J. H., et al. 1984. Evidence for a directional correspondence between eye movements and dream imagery in REM sleep. *Sleep* 7:52–63.

Ian-co, V., and P. Lavie. 1988. Patterns of eye movements and pre-eye movement alpha activity during REM sleep in sighted and blind subjects. In J. A. Horne, ed. *Sleep '88,* pp. 196–98. Stuttgart: Fischer.

Kaminer, H., and P. Lavie. 1991. Sleep and dreaming in Holocaust survivors: Dramatic decrease in dream recall in well-adjusted survivors. *Journal of Nervous and Mental Disease* 179:664–69.

Koulack, D., and D. R. Goodenough. 1976. Dream recall and dream recall failure: An arousal-retrieval model. *Psychological Bulletin* 83:975–84.

Lavie, P., and H. Kaminer. 1991. Dreams that poison sleep: Dreaming in Holocaust survivors. *Dreaming* 1:11–21.

Maury, A. 1865. *Le sommeil et les rêves: Etudes psychologiques.* Paris: Didier.

Petre-Quadens, O., H. Hussain, and C. Balaratnan. 1975. Paradoxical sleep characteristics and cultural environment: Preliminary results. *Acta Neurologica Belgica* 75:85–92.

Rechtschaffen, A. 1978. The single-mindedness and isolation of dreams. *Sleep* 1:97–109.

Vogel, G. W. 1978. Sleep-onset mentation. In A. M. Arkin, J. S. Antrobus, and

S. J. Ellman, eds. *The mind in sleep: Psychology and psychophysiology*, pp. 97–108. Hillsdale, N.J.: Erlbaum.


Chapter 9. Dreaming as a Separate Reality

Cartwright, R. 1991. Dreams that work: The relation of dream incorporation to adaptation to stressful events. *Dreaming* 1:3–9.

Cartwright, R., and L. Lamberg. 1992. *Crisis dreaming*. New York: Harper-Collins.

Castaneda, C. 1972. *The road to Ixtlan*. London: Bodley Head.

Gruber, H. E. 1981. On the relation between the "aha experiences" and the construction of ideas. *History of Science* 19:41–59.

LaBerge, S. 1985. *Lucid dreaming*. New York: Ballantine.

Lavie, P., and O. Tzischinsky. 1985. Cognitive asymmetry and dreaming: Lack of relationship. *American Journal of Psychology* 98:353–61.


Chapter 10. Do Fish Dream?

Allison, T., and D. V. Cicchetti. 1976. Sleep in mammals: Ecological and constitutional correlates. *Science* 194:732–34.

Allison, T., H. Van Twyer, and W. Goff. 1972. Electrophysiological studies of the echidna Tachyglossus aculeatus. Part 1: Waking and sleep. *Archives italiennes de biologie* 110:145–84.

Campbell, S. S., and I. Tobler. 1984. Animal sleep: A review of sleep duration across phylogeny. *Neuroscience and Bio-behavioral Reviews* 8:269–300.

Jouvet, M. 1978. Does a genetic programming of the brain occur during paradoxical sleep? In P. Buser and A. Rougeul-Buser, eds. *Cerebral correlates of conscious experience*, pp. 245–61. INSERM symposium. Amsterdam: Elsevier/North-Holland.

Kaiser, W. 1988. Busy bees need rest, too: Behavioral and electromyographical sleep signs in honeybees. *Journal of Comparative Physiology* A 163:565–84.

Karmanova, I. G. 1982. Evolution of sleep: Stages and the formation of the "wakefulness-sleep" cycle in vertebrates. Basel: Karger.

Kilduff, T. S., et al. 1993. Sleep and mammalian hibernation: Homologous adaptations and homologous processes? *Sleep* 16:372–86.

Mahowald, M. W., and C. H. Schenck. 1989. REM sleep behavior disorder. In M. H. Kryger, T. Roth, and W. C. Dement, eds. *Principles and practice of sleep medicine*, pp. 389–401. Philadelphia: Saunders.

Mukhametov, L. M. 1987. Unihemispheric slow-wave sleep in the Amazonian dolphin, Inia geoffrensis. *Neuroscience Letters* 79:128–32.

Sastre, J. P., and M. Jouvet. 1979. Le comportement onirique du chat. *Physiology and Behavior* 22:979–89.

Tobler, I. 1983. Effect of forced locomotion on the rest-activity cycle of the cockroach. *Brain Research* 8:351–60.

Vaughan, C. 1963. The development and use of an operant technique to provide evidence for visual imagery in the rhesus monkey under sensory deprivation. Ph.D. diss., University of Pittsburgh.

Zepelin, H., and A. Rechtschaffen. 1974. Mammalian sleep, longevity, and energy metabolism. *Brain Behavior and Evolution* 10:425–70.

Chapter 11. The Need for Sleep

Agnew, H. W., Jr., W. B. Webb, and R. L. Williams. 1964. The effects of stage 4 and 1-REM sleep deprivation. *Electroencephalography and Clinical Neurophysiology* 17:68–70.

Bonnet, M. H. 1991. Sleep deprivation. In M. H. Kryger, T. Roth, and W. C. Dement, eds. *Principles and practice of sleep medicine*. 2d ed., pp. 50–68. Philadelphia: Saunders.

Borbely, A. A., et al. 1981. Sleep deprivation: Effect on sleep stages and EEG power density in man. *Electroencephalography and Clinical Neurophysiology* 51:483–95.

Carskadon, M. A., and W. C. Dement. 1981. Cumulative effects of sleep restriction on daytime sleepiness. *Psychophysiology* 18:107–13.

Dement, W. C. 1976. *Some must watch while some must sleep.* San Francisco: San Francisco Book Company.

Freidmann, J., et al. 1977. Performance and mood during and after gradual sleep reduction. *Psychophysiology* 14:245–50.

Gulevich, G., W. Dement, and L. Johnson. 1966. Psychiatric and EEG observations on a case of prolonged (264 hours) wakefulness. *Archives of General Psychiatry* 15: 29–35.

Hartmann, E., F. Baekeland, and G. R. Zwilling. 1972. Psychological differences between short and long sleepers. *Archives of General Psychiatry* 26:463–68.

Johnson, I., and W. L. MacLeod. 1973. Sleep and awake behavior during gradual sleep reduction. *Perceptual and Motor Skills* 36:87–97.

Meddis, R., A. J. Pearson, and G. Langford. 1973. An extreme case of healthy insomnia. *Electroencephalography and Clinical Neurophysiology* 35:213–14.

Mitler, M. M., et al. 1988. Catastrophes, sleep, and public policy: Consensus report. *Sleep* 11:100–109.

Rechtschaffen, A., et al. 1983. Physiological correlates of prolonged sleep deprivation in rats. *Science* 221:182–84.

———. 1989. Sleep deprivation in the rat. Part 10: Integration and discussion of the findings. *Sleep* 12:68–87.

Ross, J. J. 1965. Neurological findings after prolonged sleep deprivation. *Archives of Neurology* 12:399–403.

Webb, W. B., and H. W. Agnew, Jr. 1975. The effects on subsequent sleep of an acute restriction of sleep length. *Psychophysiology* 12:367–70.

———. 1975. Are we chronically sleep-deprived? *Bulletin of the Psychonomic Society* 6:47–48.

Webb, W. B., and J. Friel. 1971. Sleep stage and personality characteristics of "natural" long and short sleepers. *Science* 171:587–88.

Wilkinson, R. T. 1968. Sleep deprivation: Performance tests for partial and selective sleep deprivation. *Progress in Clinical Psychology* 8:28–43.

Chapter 12. The Eccentricity of REM Sleep

Barbato, G., et al. 1994. Extended sleep in humans in 14-hour nights (LD 10: 14): Relationship between REM density and spontaneous awakenings. *Electroencephalography and Clinical Neurophysiology* 90:291–97.

Bloch, V., E. Hennevin, and P. Leconte. 1979. Relationship between paradoxical sleep and memory processes. In M. A. Brazier, ed. *Brain mechanisms in memory and learning,* vol. 4, pp. 329–43. New York: Raven.

Cohen, H. B., R. F. Duncan, and W. C. Dement. 1967. Sleep: The effect of electroconvulsive shock in cats deprived of REM sleep. *Science* 156:1646–48.

Crick, F., and G. Mitchison. 1983. The function of dream sleep. *Nature* 304:111–114.

Dement, W. C. 1960. The effect of dream-deprivation. *Science* 131:1705–07.

Dement, W. C., et al. 1970. A sleep researcher's odyssey: The function and clinical significance of REM sleep. In L. Madow and L. Snow, eds. *The psychodynamic implications of the physiological studies of dreams.* Springfield, Ill.: Charles C. Thomas.

Gordon, H. W., B. Frooman, and P. Lavie. 1982. Shift in cognitive asymmetries between waking from REM and non-REM sleep. *Neuropsychology* 20:99–100.

Gould, S. J. 1980. Natural selection and the human brain: Darwin vs. Wallace. In *The panda's thumb.* New York: Norton.

Greenberg, R., and E. M. Dewan. Aphasia and rapid eye movement sleep. 1969. *Nature* 223:183–84.

Jouvet, M. 1980. Paradoxical sleep and the nature-nurture controversy. *Progress in Brain Research* 53:331–46.

Karni, A., et al. 1994. Dependence on REM sleep of overnight improvement of a perceptual skill. *Science* 265:679–82.

Kleitman, N. 1982. Basic rest-activity cycle—22 years later. *Sleep* 5:311–17.

Kushida, C. A., B. M. Bergmann, and A. Rechtschaffen. 1989. Sleep deprivation in the rat. Part 4: Paradoxical sleep deprivation. *Sleep* 12:22–30.

Lavie, P. 1986. Ultrashort sleep-waking schedule. Part 3: "Gates" and "forbidden zones for sleep." *Electroencephalography and Clinical Neurophysiology* 63:414–25.

———. 1989. To nap, perchance to sleep: Ultradian aspects of napping. In D. F. Dinges and R. J. Broughton, eds. *Sleep and alertness: Chronobiological, behavioral and medical aspects of napping*, pp. 99–120. New York: Raven.

Lavie, P., A. Oksenberg, and J. Zomer. 1979. "It's time, you must wake up now." *Perceptual and Motor Skills* 49:447–50.

Lavie, P., et al. 1984. Localized pontine lesion: Nearly total absence of REM sleep. *Neurology* 34:118–20.

Parmeggiani, P. L. 1987. Interaction between sleep and thermoregulation: An aspect of the control of behavioral states. *Sleep* 10:426–35.

Phillipson, E. A. 1978. Respiratory adaptations in sleep. *Annual Review of Physiology* 40:133–156.

Ramm, P., and B. J. Frost. 1986. Cerebral and local glucose cerebral metabolism in the cat during slow wave and REM sleep. *Brain Research* 365:112–24.

Roffwarg, H. P., J. N. Muzio, and W. C. Dement. 1966. Ontogenetic development of the human sleep-dream cycle. *Science* 152:604–19.

Snyder, F. 1966. Towards an evolutionary theory of dreaming. *American Journal of Psychiatry* 123:121–36.

Vogel, G. W., et al. 1980. Improvement of depression by REM sleep deprivation. *Archives of General Psychiatry* 37:247–53.

Zepelin, H. 1986. REM sleep and the timing of self-wakenings. *Bulletin of the Psychonomic Society* 24:254–56.

Chapter 13. Sleep Centers

Akert, K., ed. 1981. *Biological order and brain organization: Selected writings of W. R. Hess*. Berlin: Springer.

Borbely, A. A., and I. Tobler. 1989. Endogenous sleep-promoting substances and sleep regulation. *Physiological Review* 69:605–70.

Bremer, G. 1935. Cerveau isolé et physiologie du sommeil. *Comptes rendus des séances de la Société de Biologie et de ses filiales* (Paris) 118:725–28.

Hess, W. R. 1965. Sleep as a phenomenon of the integral organism. In K. Akert, C. Bally, and J. P. Schade, eds. *Sleep mechanisms*. New York: Elsevier.

————. 1981. Biological order and brain organization. In K. Akert, ed. *Selected works of W. R. Hess.* Berlin: Springer.

Jouvet, M. 1967. Neurophysiology of the states of sleep. *Physiological Reviews* 47:117–77.

————. 1969. Biogenic amines and the states of sleep. *Science* 163:32–41.

Lavie, P. 1993. The sleep theory of Constantin von Economo. *Journal of Sleep Research* 2:175–78.

Lugaresi, E., et al. 1986. Fatal familial insomnia and dysautonomia with selective degeneration of thalamic nuclei. *New England Journal of Medicine* 315: 997–1003.

Magnes, J., G. Moruzzi, and O. Pompeiano. 1961. Synchronization of the EEG produced by low-frequency electrical stimulation of the region of the solitary tract. *Archives italiennes de biologie* 99:33–67.

Moruzzi, G. 1972. The sleep-waking cycle. *Ergebnisse der Physiologie, biologischen Chemie und experimentellen Pharmakologie* 64:1–165.

Moruzzi, G., and H. Magoun. 1949. Brain stem reticular formation and activation of the EEG. *Electroencephalography and Clinical Neurophysiology* 1:455.

Sacks, O. 1990. *Awakenings.* Rev. ed. London: Picador.

Sakai, K. 1988. Executive mechanisms of paradoxical sleep. *Archives italiennes de biologie* 126:259–74.

Steriade, M., and R. W. McCarley. 1990. *Brainstem control of wakefulness and sleep.* New York: Plenum.

Sterman, M. B., and C. D. Clements. 1962. Forebrain inhibitory mechanisms: Sleep patterns induced by basal forebrain stimulation in the behaving cat. *Experimental Neurology* 6:103–17.

Webb, W. B. 1978. The sleep of cojoined twins. *Sleep* 1:205–11.

von Economo, C. 1930. Sleep as a problem of localization. *Journal of Nervous and Mental Disease* 71:249–59.

Chapter 14. Sleep Medicine: The First Steps

Bixler, E. O., et al. 1979. Prevalence of sleep disorders: A survey of the Los Angeles metropolitan area. *American Journal of Psychiatry* 136:1257–62.

Coleman, R., et al. 1982. Sleep-wake disorders based upon a polysomnographic diagnosis: A national cooperative study. *Journal of the American Medical Association* 247:997–1003.

Guilleminault, G., and E. Lugaresi. 1983. Sleep/wake disorders: Natural history, epidemiology, and long-term evolution. New York: Raven.

Hauri, P. J., ed. 1991. *Case studies in insomnia.* New York: Plenum.

Hauri, P. J., and J. Fischer. 1986. Persistent psychophysiological (learned) insomnia. *Sleep* 9:38–53.

Hauri, P. J., and E. Olmsted. 1980. Childhood onset insomnia. *Sleep* 3:59–65.

Karacan, I., et al. 1976. Prevalence of sleep disturbance in a primarily urban Florida county. *Social Science and Medicine* 10:239–44.

Kryger, M. H., T. Roth, and W. Dement, eds. 1989. *Principles and practice of sleep medicine.* Philadelphia: Saunders.

Lavie, P. 1981. Sleep habits and sleep disturbances in industrial workers in Israel: Main findings and some characteristics of workers complaining of excessive daytime sleepiness. *Sleep* 4:147–58.

———. 1993. Physician education in sleep disorders: A dean of medicine's viewpoint. *Sleep* 16:760–61.

Lavie, P., et al. 1991. Sleeping under the threat of the Scud: War-related environmental insomnia. *Israel Journal of Medical Science* 27:681–86.

———. 1993. Children's sleep under the threat of attack by ballistic missiles. *Journal of Sleep Research* 2:34–37.

Munthe, A. 1975. The story of San Michele. London: John Murray.

Yourcenar, M. 1954. *The memoirs of Hadrian.* Trans. Grace Frick. New York: Farrar.

Chapter 15. Treating Insomnia

Bootzin, R. R., and P. M. Nicassio. 1978. Behavioral treatments for insomnia. In M. Hersen, R. Eissler, and P. Miller, eds. *Progress in behavior modification,* vol. 6, pp. 1–45. New York: Academic Press.

Gillin, J. C., and E. F. Byerley. 1990. The diagnosis and management of insomnia. *New England Journal of Medicine* 322:239–48.

Hauri, P. J., and S. Linde. 1990. *No more sleepless nights.* New York: Wiley.

Kales, A., M. B. Scharf, and J. Kales. 1978. Rebound insomnia: a new chemical syndrome. *Science* 201:1039–1041.

Kales, A., et al. 1974. Chronic hypnotic drug use: Ineffectiveness, drug withdrawal insomnia and dependence. *Journal of the American Medical Association* 227:511–17.

Kripke, D. F., et al. 1979. Short and long sleep and sleeping pills: Is increased mortality associated? *Archives of General Psychiatry* 36:103–16.

Mellinger, G. D., M. B. Balter, and E. H. Uhlenhuth. 1985. Insomnia and its treatment: Prevalence and correlates. *Archives of General Psychiatry* 42:225–32.

Mendelson, W. B. 1980. *The use and misuse of sleeping pills.* New York: Plenum.

Chapter 16. The Physical and Medical Causes of Insomnia

Broughton, R., and R. Baron. 1978. Sleep patterns in the intensive care unit and on the ward after acute myocardial infarction. *Electroencephalography and Clinical Neurophysiology* 45:348–60.

Coleman, R. 1982. Periodic movements in sleep (nocturnal myoclonus) and restless legs syndrome. In C. Guilleminault, ed. *Sleeping and waking disorders: Indications and techniques,* pp. 265–95. Menlo Park, Calif.: Addison-Wesley.

Feinberg, I., M. Braun, and R. L. Koresko. 1969. Stage 4 sleep in schizophrenia. *Archives of General Psychiatry* 21:262–66.

Guilleminault, C., F. L. Eldridge, and W. C. Dement. 1973. Insomnia with sleep apnea: A new syndrome. *Science* 181:856–58.

Hauri, P., and D. R. Hawkins. 1973. Alpha-delta sleep. *Electroencephalography and Clinical Neurophysiology* 34:233–37.

Kupfer, D. 1976. REM latency: A psychobiologic marker for primary depressive disease. *Biological Psychiatry* 11:159–74.

Lugaresi, E., et al. 1986. Nocturnal myoclonus and restless legs syndrome. *Advances in Neurology* 43:295–306.

Mahowald, M. W., and C. H. Schenck. 1989. REM sleep behavior disorder. In M. H. Kryger, T. Roth, and W. C. Dement, eds. *Principles and practice of sleep medicine,* pp. 389–401. Philadelphia: Saunders.

Moldofsky, H., F. A. Lue, and H. A. Smythe. 1983. Alpha EEG sleep and morning symptoms in rheumatoid arthritis. *Journal of Rheumatology* 10: 373–79.

Ohanna, N., et al. Periodic leg movements in sleep: Effect of clonazepam treatment. *Neurology* 35:408–411, 1985.

Wittig, R. M., et al. 1982. Disturbed sleep in patients complaining of chronic pain. *Journal of Nervous and Mental Disease* 170:429–31.

Zarcone, V. P., Jr., K. L. Benson, and P. A. Berger. 1987. Abnormal rapid eye movement latencies in schizophrenia. *Archives of General Psychiatry* 44:45–48.


Chapter 17. Disorders in Sleep Timing

Arendt, J., M. Aldous, and R. H. Marks. 1986. Alleviation of jet lag by melatonin: Preliminary results of controlled double blind trial. *British Medical Journal* 292:1170.

Czeisler, C. A., M. C. Moore-Ede, and R. H. Coleman. 1982. Rotating shift work schedules that disrupt sleep are improved by applying circadian principles. *Science* 217:460–63.

Czeisler, C. A., et al. 1981. Chronotherapy: Resetting the circadian clocks of patients with delayed sleep phase insomnia. *Sleep* 4:1–21.

———. 1990. Exposure to bright light and darkness to treat physiologic maladaptation to night work. *New England Journal of Medicine* 322:1253–59.

Eastman, C. 1990. Circadian rhythms and bright light: Recommendations for shift work. *Work and Stress* 4:245–60.

Knauth, P., et al. 1980. Duration of sleep depending on the type of shift work. *International Archives of Occupational and Environmental Health* 46:167–77.

Lavie, P., et al. 1989. Sleep disturbances in shift workers: A marker for maladaptation syndrome. *Work and Stress* 3:33–40.

———. 1992. Sleep-wake cycle in shift workers on a "clockwise" and "counterclockwise" rotation system. *Israel Journal of Medical Science* 28:636–44.

Monk, T. H., and S. Folkard. 1985. Individual differences in shiftwork adjustment. In Folkard and Monk, eds. *Hours of work: Temporal factors in work scheduling*, pp. 227–37. New York: Wiley.

Moore-Ede, M. C., and G. S. Richardson. 1985. Medical implications of shift work. *Annual Review of Medicine* 36:607–17.

Weitzman, E. D., et al. 1981. Delayed sleep phase syndrome: A chronobiologic disorder associated with sleep onset insomnia. *Archives of General Psychiatry* 38:737–46.

Chapter 18. Children Who Refuse to Sleep

Arkin, A. M. 1966. Sleep talking: A review. *Journal of Nervous and Mental Disease* 143:101–22.

Blatt, I., et al. 1991. The value of sleep recordings in evaluating somnambulism in young adults. *Electroencephalography and Clinical Neurophysiology* 78:407–12.

Broughton, R. J. 1968. Sleep disorders: Disorders of arousal? *Science* 159:1070–78.

Carskadon, M. A., E. D. Brown, and W. C. Dement. 1982. Sleep fragmentation in the elderly: Relationship to daytime sleep tendency. *Neurobiology of Aging* 3:321–27.

Douglas, J., and N. Richman. 1984. *My child won't sleep.* Harmondsworth: Penguin.

Ferber, R. 1985. *Solve your child's sleep problems.* New York: Simon and Schuster.

Guilleminault, C., ed. 1987. *Sleep and its disorders in children.* New York: Raven.

Haimov, I., et al. 1994. Sleep disorders and melatonin rhythms in elderly people. *British Medical Journal* 309:167.

Kavey, N. B., et al. 1990. Somnambulism in adults. *Neurology* 40:749–52.

Ophir-Cohen, M., et al. 1993. Sleep patterns of children sleeping in residential care, in Kibbutz dormitories, and at home: A comparative study. *Sleep* 16: 428–32.

Prinz, P. N., et al. 1990. Geriatrics: Sleep disorders and aging. *New England Journal of Medicine* 323:520–27.

Richman, N., et al. 1985. Behavioral methods in the treatment of sleep disorders: A pilot study. *Journal of Child Psychology and Psychiatry and Allied Disciplines* 26:581–90.

Sadeh, A., et al. 1991. Actigraphic home-monitoring of sleep-disturbed and control infants: A new method for pediatric assessment of sleep-wake patterns. *Pediatrics* 87:494–99.

Schneck, C. H., et al. 1986. Chronic behavioral disorders of human REM sleep: A new category of parasomnia. *Sleep* 9:293–306.

Chapter 19. Excessive Sleepiness, or "In the Arms of Morpheus"

Catlin, G. 1861. *The breath of life.* New York: Wiley.

Caton, R. 1889. Case of narcolepsy. *Clinical Society Transactions* 22:133–37.

Charuzi, I., et al. 1985. The effect of surgical weight reduction on sleep quality in obesity-related sleep apnea syndrome. *Surgery* 97:535–38.

Fairbanks, D. N. F., et al., eds. 1987. *Snoring and obstructive sleep apnea.* New York: Raven.

Gastaut, H., C. A. Tassinari, and B. Duron. 1966. Polygraphic study of the episodic diurnal and nocturnal (hypnic and respiratory) manifestations of the Pickwick syndrome. *Brain Research* 2:167–86.

Guilleminault, C., and M. Partinen, eds. 1990. *Obstructive sleep apnea syndrome: Clinical research and treatment.* New York: Raven.

Lavie, P. 1983. Incidence of sleep apnea in a presumably healthy working population: A significant relationship with excessive daytime sleepiness. *Sleep* 6:312–18.

———. 1984. Nothing new under the moon: Historical accounts of sleep apnea syndrome. *Archives of Internal Medicine* 144:2025–28.

———. 1987. Rediscovering the importance of nasal breathing in sleep, or shut your mouth and save your sleep. *Journal of Laryngology and Otology* 101: 558–63.

Lavie, P., R. Ben-Yosef, and A. E. Rubin. 1984. Prevalence of sleep apnea syndrome among patients with essential hypertension. *American Heart Journal* 108:373–76.

Lavie, P., N. Yoffe, I. Berger and R. Peled. 1993. The relationship between the severity of sleep apnea syndrome and 24-h blood pressure values in patients with obstructive sleep apnea. *Chest* 103:717–21.

Lugaresi, E. 1975. Snoring. *Electroencephalography and Clinical Neurophysiology* 39:59–64.

Pillar, G., and P. Lavie. 1995. Assessment of the role of inheritance in sleep apnea. *American Journal of Respiratory and Critical Care Medicine* 151: 688–91.

Sullivan, C. E., et al. 1981. Reversal of obstructive sleep apnea by continuous positive airway pressure applied through the nares. *Lancet* 1:862–65.

## Chapter 20. Narcolepsy: Reversal of the Natural Order

Aldrich, M. S. 1990. Narcolepsy. *New England Journal of Medicine.* 323:389–94.

Baker, T. L., et al. 1982. Canine model of narcolepsy: Genetic and developmental determinants. *Experimental Neurology* 75:729–62.

Critchley, M. 1962. Periodic hypersomnia and megaphagia in adolescent males. *Brain* 85:627–56.

Dement, W. C., A. Rechtschaffen, and G. Gulevich. 1966. The nature of the narcoleptic sleep attack. *Neurology* 16:18–33.

Gadoth, N., et al. 1987. Episodic hormone secretion during sleep in Kleine-Levin syndrome: Evidence for hypothalamic dysfunction. *Brain and Development* 9:309–15.

Juji, T., et al. 1984. HLA antigens in Japanese patients with narcolepsy: All patients were DR2 positive. *Tissue Antigens* 24:316–19.

Lavie, P. 1987. The "sleeping beauty": An extinguished syndrome of excessive sleepiness. *Sleep* 16:382.

———. 1991. The touch of Morpheus: Pre-20th-century accounts of sleepy patients. *Neurology* 41:1841–44.

Lavie, P., et al. 1979. Sleep patterns in Kleine-Levin syndrome. *Electroencephalography and Clinical Neurophysiology* 47:369–71.

Parkes, J. D., C. Lock, and N. Langdon. 1986. Narcolepsy and immunity. *British Medical Journal* 292:359–60.

Rechtschaffen, A., et al. 1963. Nocturnal sleep of narcoleptics. *Electroencephalography and Clinical Neurophysiology* 45:621–37.

Sacks, O. 1990. *Awakenings.* Rev. ed. London: Picador.

Wilner, A., et al. 1988. Narcolepsy-cataplexy in Israeli Jews is associated exclusively with the DR2 haplotype: A study at the serological and genomic level. *Human Immunology* 21:15–22.

# Index

Absorption rate, 180
Accidents: in sleep apnea, 228; in sleepy drivers, 49, 50, 123; in shift work, 200
Acetylcholine, 160
Acrobat's Leap experiment, 119, 121, 122
Actimeter, 7, 196, 197
Active sleep, 21, 29
Advanced sleep phase syndrome, 192
*Adventures of Don Quixote, The*, 174
African-Americans, 237
Aging, sleep quality of, 30
Agnew, B., 115, 117
Alcmaeon, 2
Alcohol, 176, 177
Algae, ix
Alpha-delta sleep, 185
Altschule, M., 61
Amobarbital, 178
"Anemia," 4
Anorexia nervosa, 240
Antidepressants, 188
Anxiety, 168, 171, 173, 181
Aristotle, 3, 151
Aschoff, J., xii, 42, 56
Aserinsky, E., 17, 19, 29, 124, 148, 159
Automatism, 208
Autonomic nervous system, 129, 151, 242
*Awakenings*, 151, 240

Barbiturates, 178, 179
Beck, A., 8
Bed-rocking, 209

Bedwetting, 209
Benzodiazepines, 177, 178
Berger, H., 9, 12, 154
Biofeedback, 12, 175
Biological clocks, 189, 193, 203, 207; and light-dark, 54–55; in infants, 36; history of, 55–56; in animals, 59–60; in body temperature, 57–59; light entrainment, 60. *See also* Biological rhythms, Circadian rhythm, Sleep-wakefulness rhythm
Biological rhythms, 161
Blind, 63, 190
Bloch, V., 138
Blood gas levels, 129
Body movements, 7, 27
Body temperature, 57, 195; Aschoff's studies, 42–43; early recordings of, 57; in time-free environment, 58
Boehringer Ingelheim, xii
Bonaparte, Napoleon, 114
Brain centers, degeneration of, 186
Brain injury, 142
Brain mechanisms, in sleep, 154–160; of temperature regulation, 127, 130. *See also* Brain stem, Hypothalamus, Pons, Raphe nuclei, Sleep center, Thalamus
Brain Research Institute (Los Angeles), 159
Brain stem, 143, 154, 156, 157, 159, 160
Brain stimulation, 155
Brain "thermostat," 127
Brain waves: alpha, 12; beta, 12; delta, 16–17; during falling asleep, 13; in

Brain waves (*continued*)
  REM, 22; in wakefulness, 11; K-
  complex, 15–16; lab recordings of,
  10–11; spindles, 15; theta, 13, 219
*Breath of Life, The*, 226, 227
Bremer, F., 154, 158, 159
Bright light, 194
Broughton, R., 211
Burning-light culture, 121
Burwell, S., 223
Bush, George, 244

Cancer, 185
Carbohydrates, 177
Carskadon, M., 50, 117
Cartwright, R., 94
Castaneda, C., 92
Cataplexy, 234
Catlin, G., 225, 226
Caton, R., 8, 223
Cats, 107, 158
Cerebral arousal, 135, 146
Cerebrum, 153
Cervantes, 173
Chamomile, 177
Charcot, J. M., 172
Chernobyl, 199
Chester Beatty papyrus, 89
Chicago, University of, 18, 20, 69,
  124
*Children's Sleep*, 6, 7
Chronic fatigue, 185
Chronic pain, 185
Chronobiology, 54. *See also* Biological
  clocks
Chronotherapy, 193
Circadian rhythm, 41
Clonazepam, 185
Coffee, 176
Convulsion threshold, 136
Cortisol, 32
CPAP (continuous positive air
  pressure), 231, 233

Crick, F., 141, 143, 144
Czeisler, C., 59

Dagan, Y., 84
Darwin, C., 147
Death, because of sleep deprivation,
  126–127
Delayed sleep phase, 190
Delayed sleep phase syndrome,
  treatment of, 193–194
Delphi, 65
Dement, W., xii, 20, 21, 68, 85, 120,
  121, 132, 134, 136, 145, 146, 159,
  227, 236
Dementia, 144, 186
Depression, 135, 186, 187
*De rerum natura*, 6
Descartes, R., 61
*De somno et vigilia*, 3
d'Hervey de Saint Denis, 94
Diabetics, 184
Dickens, C., 224, 225
DNA, 141, 144
Dogs, 236
DR2 antigen, 237
Dreaming: and controlling reality, 92–
  93; and creativity, 89–92; and eye-
  movements, 85–88; during Gulf War,
  72–73; early and late REM, 68;
  effects of external stimuli, 79–90;
  effects of trauma on, 81–85; in
  animals, 106–110; in non-REM
  stages, 70, 72; in sleep lab, 73–75; of
  the blind, 86–87; of Holocaust
  survivors, 82–84; of Mr. R., 94–97;
  war-related post-traumatic, 84–85;
  recall of, 80–81; repression of, 84;
  significance of, 65; single-
  mindedness of, 79; sources of, 70,
  72–75
Dreams: about sheep, 74–75; of a
  Holocaust survivor, 81–82; of a
  monkey, 106; of a narcoleptic, 235;

of Eskimo, 95; of Guillotine, 78; of
Kekule, 90; about ping-pong, 85;
post-traumatic, 81
Dream smile, 109
Drug tolerance, 172. *See also*
Benzodiazepines, Barbiturates,
Sleeping pills

Echidna, 103
Economo, C. von, 5, 151–155, 170,
240
Edison, T., ix, 114
Einstein, A., 114
Electric shock, 136, 139
Electric shock treatment, 137
Electrical stimulation, 157, 158, 170
Electroencephalogram, 8; history of, 8–
9. *See also* Brain waves
Encephalitis lethargica, 5, 151. *See also*
Sleeping sickness, Economo, C. von
Endocrinology, 31
Endymion, 239
Enuresis, 211
Epilepsy, 234
Epimenides, 239
Erling-Andachs, 42
Excessive sleepiness, 153, 217; causes
of, 218; in early literature, 216
Eye movements, and dream story, 87; at
sleep onset, 14; density of, 187; in
lucid dreams, 93; in REM, 22;
muscle control of, 24

Falling asleep: conditioning of, 169–
170; physiological changes, 13
Fatal insomnia, 156
Fear of sleep, 169
Fetal movements, 30
Florida, University of, xii, 44, 133
Fluids theory, 31
Food and Drug Administration (U.S.),
179
"Forbidden zone" for sleep, xi, 50–53

Foulkes, D., 69
Frederick I (Barbarossa), 239
Freud, S., 66, 70, 77

Galen, 3, 31, 151
Galvani, L., 8
Gardner, R., 120, 121
Gelineau, J., 235
Girl of Montrose, The, 240
Giora, Z., xi
Gonadotropines, 33, 242
Gonen, A., 117
Gould, S. J., 147
Greek medicine, 31
Greek mythology, 2
Greenberg, R., 139
Gross, M., 79
Growth hormone, 32
Grunstein, R., 232
*Guinness Book of Records, The*, 120
Gulf War, 71, 165, 167, 168

Haifa, 72, 166
Haimov, I., 213, 214
Half-life, of sleeping drugs, 180
Hallucinations, 118–119
Hartmann, E., 113
Harvard University, 11, 59, 144, 147,
224
Headaches, 185
Heat corridor, 127
Heath, C., 225
Hebrew University, 158
Hennevin, E., 138
Hess, W. R., 155, 156
Hibernation, 103, 240
Hippocampus, 138
Hippocrates, 31, 55
Hobson, A., 144
Holocaust, 81
Homer, 2
Honda, Y., 239
Horne, J., 114

Hypertension, 229
Hypnagogic hallucinations, 70, 77, 235
"Hypnic jerk," 14
Hypnogram, 26
Hypnos, 2, 178
Hypnotoxins, 4, 153
Hypothalamus, 153, 155, 157, 158, 170, 242
Hypothermia, 126

*Iliad*, 2
Infants, 28, 35
Insomnia, 163–164; conditioning of, 170; causes of, 163–164; chronic, 169–173, 182; definition of, 163; in mental disorders, 186–188; primary, 173; situational, 165, 168, 169; subjective and objective, 171–172; treatment of, 161, 174–175; war-related, 165–166
Intensive care, 185
*Interpretation of Dreams, The*, 66, 78
"Inverted pot" technique, 135
Israel, 73, 121, 165, 168, 202, 237, 242
Israel Defense Forces, 122

Japan, 199, 238
Jena Psychiatric Hospital, 9
Jet lag, 200–204; direction effect of, 203; signs of, 201; treatment of, 203–204
Jewish daily prayer book, 2
Joe (Dickens's "fat boy"), 224, 225, 226
Jouvet, M., x, xii, 70, 86, 107, 109, 136, 159, 160, 243

K-complex, 26
Kaminer, H., 82
Karni, A., 140
Kekule, F. A. von, 90, 91, 146
Kidney disease, 184
King Arthur, 239

Kitay, J., 61
Klein, E., 168
Kleine, W., 240
Kleine-Levin syndrome, 240–242
Kleitman, N., xii, 5, 17, 29, 68, 120, 124, 147, 159; life story of, 18–19; infant study by, 36
Kramer, M., 85
Kripke, D., xi, 161, 179, 219
Kronauer, R., 59

L-dopa, 152, 240
La Salpêtrière, 173
Laberge, S., 93
Lady Macbeth, 209
Lebanon war, 84
Leconte, P., 138
Leg movements, 213
Lerner, A., 61
*Le sommeil et les rêves*, 77
Levin, M., 240
Lewy, A., 62
Light treatment, 194
Light-dark cycle, 189
Long-term memory, 137, 139
Lucid dreaming, 93–94
Lucretius, 6
Lugaresi, E., 156
Lyons, University of (France), 159

*Macbeth*, 175, 210
Magnes, Y., 158
Magoun, H., 157, 158, 159
Mahowald, M., 109
Maimonides, 111
Mairan J. de, 55
Mammoth Cave (Kentucky), 19
Maury, A., 76
McCarley, B., 144
Meddis, R., 112
Melatonin, 60, 61–64, 194, 213; light's effect on, 62; treatment with, 214. *See also* Pineal gland

*Mémoires d'Hadrien*, 163
Memory consolidation, 138, 139
Metabolic rate, 127
Midnight Cave (Texas), 42
"Milky Ways," 36
Missile attacks, 165
Mitchison, G., 141, 143
Montefiore Hospital (New York), 193,
    238
More, T., 111
Morrison, A., 107
Mortality, 229
Moruzzi, G., 157, 158
Mukhametov, L., xii, 103
Multiple sleep latency test (MSLT), 50,
    117
Munthe, A., 173
Muscle tonus, 11

Nap, 50, 171, 214
Narcolepsy, 25, 161, 226, 234; first
    description of, 235; in dogs, 236; in
    Jews, 237–238; genetics of, 237–238;
    prevalence of, 238–239; treatment of,
    239
Nasal breathing, 226
*Nature*, 141
Navy, U.S., 115, 121
Nazis, 9, 81
Nerve stimulation, 8
Nervous legs syndrome, 184. *See also*
    Periodic leg movements
Neural network theory, 141
*Neurology*, 142
New York, 200, 201
Nicotine, 176
Nightmares, 142
Night terrors, 209, 211
Night work, 195. *See also* Shift
    work
Nobel Prize, 5, 155, 141
"Nodding off," 13
Nonrestorative sleep, 185

Noradrenalin, 160
Nursing homes, 214

Ogier (national hero of Denmark),
    239
Oksenberg, A., 148
"One-eyed" sleep, 100
Owls, 190

*Panda's Thumb, The*, 147
Paradoxical sleep, 21, 99, 101; and
    instinctual behavior, 136–137;
    deprivation of, 127–128, 136–137; in
    dolphin, 105; rebound of, 128;
    without atonia, 107–108. *See also*
    REM sleep
Parasomnia, 211
Parkinson's disease, 152
Pavlov, I., 5
Pearlman, C., 139
Penile erections, 25, 129
Pentobarbital, 178
Periodic leg movements, 184, 185. *See
    also* Nervous legs syndrome
Perrault, C., 240
Petre Quadens, O., 87
Pharmaceutical companies, 161, 179
Phillipson, E., 148
"Phlegm," 31
Phototherapy, 193
Pickwickian syndrome, 226
*Pickwick Papers, The*, 224
Pieron, H., 124, 125, 153
Pineal gland, 61, 157. *See also*
    Melatonin
Pituitary gland, 33
Plato, 3, 151
Polysomnographic recordings, 11
Pons, 143, 157. *See also* Brain stem
Post-traumatic recovery, 185
Prolactin, 242
Prolonged sleep, 239–240
Proust, M., 171

Psychoses, 186
Pulsatile, 34

Raphe nuclei, 160
Rapid eye movement. *See* REM
Rats, 126, 138
Rechtschaffen, A., xii, 79, 124, 125, 128, 135, 146
Relaxation techniques, 175
REM, 5, 19, 21, 23, 59, 74, 115, 124, 147, 156, 212, 244; across night, 29; after CPAP, 232; and cortisol secretion, 33; and dreaming, 66–68; and instincts, 109–110; and memory, 137–142; as "gate" from sleep, 148; awakening from, 67, 75, 148–149; brain mechanisms of, 143, 159–160; sleeping pills' effect on, 179; in aphasics, 140; in birds, 100; in depression, 135, 137; in infants, 29, 148; in mental retardation, 142; in narcoleptics, 236; in primitive tribes, 87–88; nearly total absence of, 142–145; need of, 131–132; ontogenetic theory, 146; physiological characteristics, 22–23; physiological changes, 129–131; roles of, 145–150; similarities with wakefulness, 147–148; temperature regulation in, 130. *See also* Paradoxical sleep
REM behavior disorder, 212
REM density, 187
REM deprivation, and learning, 140–142; and arousal, 135–137; and perceptual learning, 141; first human study, 132–133; methods of, 131; therapeutic effects of, 137
*Remembrance of Things Past*, 171
REM latency, 27; in depression, 187; in psychoses, 186
Respiratory control system, 130, 148
Respiratory disorders, 184, 218, 219
Reticular formation, 158

Rheumatic ailments, 184, 185
Rhombencephalon, 158
Richman, Naomi, 208
Right hemisphere, 149
Rigler, L., xii
Rip van Winkle, 152, 239
Road accidents, 49
*Road to Ixtlan, The*, 92
Roffwarg, H., 146
Rooney, A. (journalist), 213
Royal Academy of Science (Paris), 55

Sacks, O., 151, 152, 240
Sadeh, A., 208
Sagi, D., 140
Sanctorius, S., 57
San Diego, xi, 115, 116, 121, 161, 179, 219
Schenk, C., 109
Schizophrenia, 142, 152, 186
*Science*, 21,132
Secobarbital, 178
Serotonin, 160, 243
Shakespeare, 210
Shift rota, 199
Shift work, 195, 196; accidents during, 200; during nineteenth century, 199; planning of, 199
Short-term memory, 137
Siamese twins, 153
Siesta, 50
Siffre, M., 42
"Silent channel," 168
Sleep: and hormonal secretions, 32–33; as death, 2; awakening at predetermined time, 148; in birds, 99–101; during eighteenth and nineteenth centuries, 4; in Greek philosophy, 3; in insects, 99; in mammals, 101–103; during Renaissance, 3; in reptiles, 99; of antelopes, 102; of bears, 102; of dolphins, 103–105; of shift workers,

195; passive state, 2; role of, 124–
128; shortest recorded, 111–112;
stage *1*, 13, 14; stage *2*, 16; stage *4*,
17, 23; vasomotor theories, 4
*Sleep and Wakefulness*, 18, 36
Sleep apnea, 187, 219; complaints of,
221–222; dreams of, 79–80; gender
relation, 223; history of, 223–228;
physicians' disbelief, 227–228;
recordings of, 210–220; REM sleep
in, 232; risks of, 228–230; stage *3–4*
in, 232; treatment of, 230–233; types
of, 222. *See also* Pickwickian
syndrome
Sleep assessment, 5–6
Sleep automatism, 212. *See also*
Parasomnia
Sleep center, 153
Sleep "clock," 47, 53, 59
Sleep deprivation: and heat loss, 127;
consequences of, 118; in army, 119;
in rats, 125–128; in record books,
120–121; "psychosis" of, 119
Sleep disorders, causes of, 162; in
children, 205; in elderly, 212–215;
in industrial workers, 217. *See also*
Insomnia, Narcolepsy, Parasomnia,
Sleep apnea
Sleep "gate," 50–53, 90, 148–149, 194
Sleep habits, change of, 114–117; in
children, 192; in military, 121–123;
in residential homes, 206; industry
workers, 111; of physicians, 123
Sleepiness, 116
Sleeping Beauty, 239, 240
Sleeping drugs, 178–183, 244. *See also*
Sleeping pills
"Sleeping Effie," 240
Sleeping partner, 208
Sleeping pills, 172; choice of, 180;
effects of, 172–173; in elderly, 214;
rules of use, 181; withdrawal from,
182

Sleeping sickness, 151–153, 240. *See
also* Encephalitis lethargica
Sleep need, 112–113
Sleep paralysis, 23–24, 235
Sleep "propensity," 52
Sleep rituals, 205, 207
Sleep stages, cycle of: 26; in adults, 30;
in elderly, 30
Sleep talking, 209
*Sleep, the Gentle Tyrant*, 113
Sleep timing, 189
Sleep-wakefulness rhythm, after a flight,
202; Andachs's studies, 43;
disruption of, 46; erratic in normal
environment, 48–49; in caves, 42; in
infants, 39; in isolation, 40–46;
longer than twenty-four hours, 189; of
a shift worker, 198; Webb's study, 44–
46. *See also* Advanced sleep phase
syndrome, Delayed sleep phase
syndrome
Sleepwalking, 107, 186, 209–210
Slow eye movements, 20
Smith, E., 56
Smoking, 176
Snoring, 221, 226
Snyder, F., 67, 148
*Some Must Watch While Some Must
Sleep*, 85, 120
Somnambulism, 210
Stage 3–4: and automatism, 211; and
depression, 135; and growth
hormone, 32; awakening from, 149;
effects of sleeping pills, 179
Stanford Sleep Laboratory, 93
Stanford University, 236
Sterman, B., 169
Stevenson, R. L., 90
*Story of San Michele, The*, 173
*Strange Case of Dr. Jekyll and Mr.
Hyde, The*, 90
"Strong" oscillator, 59
Sullivan, C., 231

"Sun" clock, 46
"Sunday night insomnia," 177
Szymanski, 7

Takahashi, 32
Takao, J., 239
Tartini, G., 90
Technion Sleep Laboratory, xii, 10,
    47, 51, 82, 87, 94, 111, 142,
    164, 167, 178, 184, 186, 189,
    195, 228, 230, 231, 234, 237,
    240.
Teeth grinding, 211
Tel Aviv, 29, 72, 166, 200, 201
Tel Aviv University, xi, 23
Telekinesis, 9
Telepathy, 9
Thalamus, 156, 157
Thanatos, 2
Thebes, 89
Theta waves, 220
Three Mile Island, 200
Time-free environment, 41, 46
Time cues, 41
Tobler, I., xii, 101
Toronto, University of, 148
Tracheostomy, 227, 230
Trillo del Diavolo, 91
Trip, P., 120
Tzischinsky, O., 64

University of California, Los Angeles,
    169
Ultrashort sleep-wake cycle (7/13), 51
Unihemispheric sleep, 105
Union Carbide, 200. See also Dreaming,
    of Mr. R.

Vigilant sleep, 100
Violent awakening, 109. See also REM
    behavior disorder
Vogel, G., 135
Voltaire, 173

Wakefulness center, 157–158
Wallace, A. R., 147
Watson, J., 141
Weak oscillator, 59
Webb, W. B., xi, 2, 36, 44, 113, 115,
    117, 245
Wehr, T., 149
Weight reduction, 231
Weitzman, E., 193
Wyoming, University of, 70

Yourcenar, M., 163, 165

Zion, Libby, 123
Zomer, J., 148
Zurich, University of, 79, 101
Zurich Physiological Institute, 155